# PUBLISHING THE DNP PROJECT

# PUBLISHING THE DNP PROJECT

AN EVIDENCE-BASED APPROACH

DIANE B. MONSIVAIS, FRANCHESCA E. NUNEZ, AND LESLIE K. ROBBINS

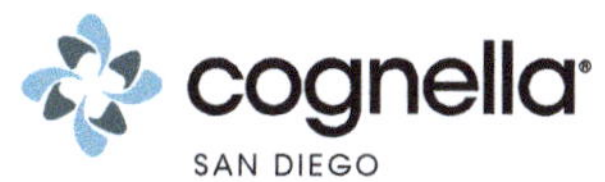

cognella®
SAN DIEGO

Bassim Hamadeh, CEO and Publisher
Amanda Martin, Executive Publisher
Amy Smith, Senior Project Editor
Jeanine Rees, Production Editor
Emely Villavicencio, Senior Graphic Designer
Kylie Bartolome, Licensing Specialist
Natalie Piccotti, Director of Marketing
Kassie Graves, Senior Vice President, Editorial



Cover image copyright © 2022 iStockphoto LP/Roni Nurdiansyah.
Cover image copyright © 2019 iStockphoto LP/malija.
Cover image copyright© 2019 iStockphoto LP/OZANKUTSAL.

Printed in the United States of America.

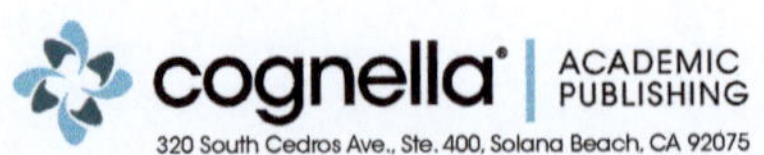

320 South Cedros Ave., Ste. 400, Solana Beach, CA 92075

# BRIEF CONTENTS

# DETAILED CONTENTS

# REVIEWERS

Dr. Mariya Tankimovich, DNP, APRN, CRNP, FNP-C, CNE
Pennsylvania State University

Kathleen S. Jordan, DNP, RN, FNP-BC, ENP-C, SANE-P, FAEN, FAANP
Clinical Professor
The University of North Carolina at Charlotte

Jeffery Ramirez, PhD, PMHNP, CNE, CARN-AP, FNAP, FAANP, FAAN
Gonzaga University, School of Health Sciences

Jane A. Tiedt, PhD, RN, ANEF
Gonzaga University, School of Health Sciences, Spokane, WA

James Papesca, DNP, APRN, CRNA
Assistant Professor of Nursing
Regis College
Young School of Nursing
Weston, Massachusetts

Heather Moore, DNP, MSN, BSN, RN, CNL
Xavier University

Dr. Edmund Travers, DNP, MSN, RN
Regis College
Massachusetts

Celeste Mulry Baldwin, PhD, MS, APRN, CNS
Regis College, Young School of Nursing
Online DNP Program
Weston, MA

Laureen M. Donovan
Shepherd University

Kathryn Niemeyer, PhD, MSc, MSN, FNP-BC, RN
Ferris State University, College of Health Professions, School of
Nursing

# CHAPTER 1

# Introduction to Publishing for DNP-Prepared Faculty

When Expectations Clash With Reality—
Publishing Your DNP Project

## Objectives

- Describe the importance of publishing DNP projects for the nursing discipline.
- Explore challenges faced by DNP-prepared faculty who are expected to publish.
- Provide an overview of the book.

## Key Terms

- **DNP project:** A clinical scholarly project carried out at the end of a DNP program.
- **Academic publishing:** Dissemination of academic scholarship.

## Opening Scenario

Dr. Emily Avila had been so excited when she started her new role as a full-time College of Nursing faculty member. She'd just been awarded her DNP degree, and after many years in clinical practice, she was anxious to share her clinical expertise with students. Her experiences as a preceptor had always been one of the most fulfilling parts of her job, and the positive feedback from students convinced her that teaching was what she was meant to do. When the opportunity to be a full-time faculty member was offered to her, she readily accepted.

To Dr. Avila's dismay, the transition from practice to academia wasn't quite as smooth as she expected. Her clinical expertise was only a tiny portion of what she needed to know, and she found she was embarrassed about having to ask a seemingly endless stream of questions. The multiple skills involved in transitioning to the faculty role had surprised (and somewhat scared) her. Not only did the role involve teaching, but also course and curriculum development (and ongoing revision), evaluating learning, and interacting with a dizzying array of personalities in both faculty and students. She'd always been able to develop excellent working relationships with students when she was a preceptor, but now she found she doubted her ability to develop that kind of relationship with a whole class at once. On top of that, one of her fellow faculty members had not been especially welcoming when they met, and Dr. Avila wondered if she had done something to offend her new colleague. The myriad of other responsibilities associated with her academic appointment, such as committee work, faculty meetings, service expectations, and maintaining her certification through practice, left her feeling overwhelmed and a little helpless.

Dr. Avila has now been informed that she was expected to mentor DNP students to publish their DNP project reports. She had never published anything, and if she were honest with herself, she'd have to admit the whole idea of publishing was somewhat terrifying, as well as puzzling. She was simply unsure of the reasons anyone would put themselves through the aggravation and intense work involved when there seemed to be so little reward (and perhaps even punishment) for doing so. One of her classmates had submitted a manuscript and been rejected immediately. He shared with everyone the feedback had been humiliating. Dr. Avila wasn't anxious to have the same experience and readily became frustrated at the thought of having to mentor a student through a process she didn't understand herself.

She found that being placed in the role of a novice made her acutely uncomfortable and produced a level of fear and anxiety she hadn't experienced since her 1st year in clinical practice. She longed for her old job when she was the expert that everyone sought out with their questions. How would she ever figure it all out? She sought out her mentor, Dr. Esperanza Duran, to let her know she may have made a mistake in taking the job, as she felt completely unqualified for the position.

Dr. Duran nodded understandingly and began by saying, "Do you remember your first year as a nurse practitioner? Chances are, you felt overwhelmed then too. You were learning to manage your time when seeing patients, and you probably checked and rechecked your plan of care and prescriptions multiple times to make sure they were correct. At the same time, you were learning about the clinic system and the people you worked with. No doubt you took at least twice as long to get things done as your more experienced colleagues. As you found colleagues who guided you in the new role and attended professional development activities, your confidence built slowly. Transitioning to the role of a faculty member can also be a slow process. And publishing is part of that role. We'll talk about the details in the future, but for now, consider the professional and personal rewards that publishing brings with it. Career advancement, being recognized as a subject matter expert, expanding your network, and contributing to nursing's body of knowledge are all very important. Please give yourself permission to be a beginner as you learn a new role and transition into it. Your confidence will build through working with colleagues who are anxious to assist you and by attending professional development activities." Dr. Duran asks Dr. Avila to answer some questions that will help her think about academic writing, and Dr. Avila agrees.

# When Expectations Clash With Reality

The chance for DNP-prepared nurses to collectively make a difference in nursing practice through publishing their DNP projects has never been greater. With enrollment in DNP programs almost twice that of PhD programs (Anderson et al., 2019), the volume of evidence being generated from DNP projects is extensive. When salient and valid project outcomes about health care costs, patient outcomes, and quality and safety initiatives are published, practitioners are then able to build a body of evidence to inform and improve care globally. The benefit to nursing practice, and health care in general, is undeniable.

However, the skills needed to transform a DNP project report into a publication-worthy manuscript are under-recognized and underappreciated. While the benefits of mentorship for scholarly productivity are well established (Cleary et al., 2023; Dunlap et al., 2023), faculty are often unprepared to effectively mentor students in publication (Anderson et al., 2019; Smeltzer et al., 2014). Traditionally, PhD faculty have been guided in publication during their academic programs or hold positions for which publication is a requirement for promotion and tenure. They are, therefore, more familiar with the process of publishing and better able to guide students. Research shows that a higher number of nursing doctoral graduates publish their work when a PhD-prepared faculty mentor serves as a chair on the committee as compared to DNP-prepared faculty (Anderson et al., 2019).

The expectations for publishing the DNP project vary widely among DNP programs, and only 10.7% of programs in a national survey (214 projects from 120 schools) included the DNP roadmap element of a traditional journal article planned or completed (Milner et al., 2023). Some programs require students to submit a journal manuscript in order to graduate but provide no guidance on following up after the manuscript is reviewed. Peer reviewers spend hours providing feedback for revision, yet the newly graduated author has no intention of revising the work. Clearly, the practice of requiring a submission without guidance contributes to the already overburdened manuscript peer-review system. Yet, it hardly seems fair to ask already overburdened faculty to assume an ongoing mentorship role with students who have graduated. Who, then, should be providing the mentorship for publishing? If the newly hired DNP faculty member is fortunate, they will be assigned a scholarship mentor who can provide guidance.

We know firsthand the challenges facing a faculty member during the publishing process can be significant. High teaching loads and university service requirements, in addition to family commitments, create a continual time crunch. Adding manuscript development to the mix is usually unrealistic. But with strong guidance and mentorship, it can be possible.

Because you can't effectively mentor anyone in what you don't know, the purpose of this book is to share evidence-based approaches for developing publishing competencies of DNP-prepared faculty. This book is meant to guide you through the process. You'll have the steps and resources needed to create a publication-worthy manuscript from your own DNP project report and those of your future students.

In each chapter, you'll find exemplars, stories, evidence-based content and resources, and application exercises so that you can test out what you are learning (and help you retain the information). An unfolding case study that follows a novice faculty member will demonstrate the process using easily relatable situations.

## Introduction to the Authors

As mid- to late-career-level academics in a college of nursing, we're part of the teaching team in a DNP program. Our academic appointments include the mandate that we publish, so we've had publishing experience that we've been able to share both informally and formally with colleagues. We'll take you through some of our own experiences with academic writing and working with DNP students and faculty colleagues. Those experiences led to our reasons for writing this book, which provides a guide for DNP-prepared faculty who are expected to mentor DNP students to publication but have not published themselves. Using a friendly conversational style, each chapter is set up to follow the principles of neuro-education using the brain targeted teaching model (Hardimann, 2012) as the framework. Research shows this approach can enhance learning through strengthening or creating new neuronal connections. It sounds daunting, but don't worry; you'll find it very user-friendly.

The book is based on the premise that the reader is a relatively recent DNP graduate with a completed DNP project report. The project report can be used to develop skills in publication, which can then be used to mentor future students. While the topics covered certainly have commonalities with other forms of scholarly publication (e.g., creating manuscripts from a dissertation), the focus is intended for the DNP-prepared faculty member or clinician. Although the focus of this book is on postmaster's DNP programs for advanced practice registered nurses, the information is also applicable to other programs, including postmaster's DNP programs for leadership and BSN to DNP programs. All DNP programs meet the same essentials and have a final or capstone project with dissemination of the project information an important goal for graduates upon program completion and throughout their careers. Since the information is presented in a format that allows readers to select and use applicable sections, it is appropriate for a variety of learners, including students and DNP program faculty and mentors.

The time and energy challenges that come with writing a manuscript may make you feel overwhelmed. That's a common reaction! We hope the step-by-step guidance provided in this book will equip you with the confidence and skills needed to start overcoming the challenges. Academic writing is not only about skills such as structuring sentences, knowing grammar and punctuation rules, or developing your central idea. Academic writing also involves managing your emotions and your routines, which are skills you no doubt already use daily. And learning the publication process will be reinforced by neuroeducational principles that are incorporated in each chapter.

Neuroeducation represents the intersection of neuroscience, psychology, and education research and how that research can be used to improve teaching and learning practices (American Psychological Association, Dictionary of Psychology, 2018).

Linking new learning to what you already know is a key neuroeducational principle, since our brains filter new information through the lens of prior experiences. That's why your DNP project report will be your starting point. You know your project well and can link your experiences with it to new concepts about publishing.

The chapters are designed to give you the background and approaches needed to be successful in publishing your DNP project, and then in guiding your students to publish their own projects. The book takes you through chapters dealing with pathways to successful writing, faculty–student coauthorship, unleashing the publication potential of your project, finding a journal for your manuscript, using peer reviewing to improve authorship skills, and a look at the future of academic communications. So that you can quickly get an idea of what is included in the book, summaries of each chapter follow.

# Chapter 2: Pathways to Successful Writing

Writing in the nursing discipline is complex, even within a specific category of writing. We'll focus on academic writing in the context of DNP project reports and the nuances in that category. Our shared educational and health care experiences as nurses allow all of us to understand that there is a relationship between our disciplinary values and writing.

Nursing's professional values call for scholarly inquiry and dissemination (American Nurses Association, 2015), yet the emotional toll required to carry out those activities is often under-recognized. Frustration looms large in just about any writing project for most academic writers because it's simply part of the process and the human experience (Sword et al., 2018). The temptation to give up is strong if you don't have a mentor who can coach you through those frustrating times.

## Chapter 3: Caution! Faculty-Student Coauthorship

Coauthorship can be difficult terrain to navigate, even for experienced authors. However, for early career DNP faculty who would like to coauthor with students, it can be filled with potential landmines that often explode unexpectedly. Specific strategies and tools for successful and ethical coauthorship with former students are essential to protect both parties from detonating a landmine.

## Chapter 4: Unleashing the Publication Potential of Your DNP Project Report

Your DNP project report is a product of your persistence and commitment, and it got you to the graduation finish line. Your report showed that you were able to meet requirements, but those are quite different than manuscript requirements. It will take some rethinking and rearranging of your project report to turn it into a manuscript. A worksheet to help you create a manuscript "slant" is the first step. Although this may take some time, a well-crafted worksheet will provide substantial benefits as you revise your project report.

## Chapter 5: Finding a Journal for Your Manuscript-in-Progress

Your manuscript deserves to be published in a trustworthy journal. Differentiating between trustworthy journals and predatory journals is the first step. We'll take you through the process of targeting appropriate journals for your work. Like any other skill, it takes some practice!

## Chapter 6: Improving Authorship Skills Through Peer Reviewing

As an author, you expect peer reviewers to be available to provide feedback that strengthens your work. When you reverse the role and become a peer reviewer, you'll find that providing helpful critiques to others may help you more quickly notice ways to improve your own writing. Peer reviewing, therefore, is a valuable service to the profession that also provides benefits to you as an author. Resources for developing peer-reviewing skills are plentiful, and we'll share some with you.

## Chapter 7: Looking Toward the Future of Academic Communication

What kind of publishing competencies will you need for your future in academia? No prediction is perfect, but we'll summarize current thinking.

## Reflection Exercises

Think about your own experiences with writing and publishing. While you may not have published your academic work, you no doubt have heard it discussed. Were the discussions generally positive or negative? How does that affect your wish to publish?

The following questions are examples taken directly from the complete Situated Academic Writing Self-Efficacy Scale (Mitchell et al., 2021, p. 17). Use your writing experiences in your DNP program to answer the questions.

1. When I write, I can think about my audience and write so they clearly understand my meaning.

2. When I receive feedback on my writing, no matter how it makes me feel, I can use that feedback to improve my writing in the future.

3. When I reflect on what I am writing I can make my writing better.

4. When I read articles about my topic, the connections I feel with the ideas of other authors can inspire me to express my own ideas in writing.

5. When I look at the overall picture I've presented in my writing, I can assess how all the pieces tell the complete story of my topic or argument.

6. I can recognize when I've wandered away from writing what my audience needs to know and have begun writing about interesting, but unrelated, ideas.

7. With each new writing assignment, I can adapt my writing to meet the needs of that assignment.

8. When I seek feedback on my writing, I can decide when that feedback should be ignored or incorporated into a revision in my writing.

9. I can use creativity when writing an academic paper.

10. I feel I can give my writing a creative spark and still sound professional.

11. I feel I can develop my own writing voice (ways of speaking in my writing that are uniquely me).

12. Even with very specific assignment guidelines, I can find ways of writing my assignment to make it original or unique.

## Closing Scenario

Dr. Avila follows up with her mentor and says, "I'm beginning to understand how important publishing is and about some of the challenges. The self-assessment questions really got me thinking more deeply about how complicated writing can be."

She highlighted one area that especially stood out for her. As she reflected on her DNP program, she remembered the feelings of confusion she sometimes felt with feedback from different instructors. Some focused on APA format; others on the content and structure of the paper. Even within the same course, the range of feedback was highly variable. She realized that it was the substantive feedback (instead of formatting feedback) that helped her develop her ideas and central concepts, as well as improve the structure of the paper for improved readability. She said she was puzzled about what it meant to be creative within the constraints of an academic paper. "You've given this some excellent thought," her mentor assured her. As we move through the writing process, we'll delve more deeply into those issues and more.

## End of Chapter Questions

1. Why is it important to publish DNP project outcomes?

2. What are some challenges faculty who publish their academic writing face?

3. Which questions from the Situated Academic Writing Self-Efficacy Scale (Mitchell et al., 2021) were noteworthy for you? Noteworthy might mean you had never thought about the item before reading it on the survey or it reminded you of an experience related to your writing as a student.

## References

American Nurses Association. (2015). Code of ethics for nurses with interpretive statements (2nd ed.). American Nurses Publishing

American Psychological Association, Dictionary of Psychology. (2018, April 4). *Neuroeducation*. https://dictionary.apa.org/neuroeducation

Anderson, K. M., McLaughlin, M. K., Crowell, N. A., Fall-Dickson, J. M., White, K. A., Heitzler, E. T., Kesten, K. S., & Yearwood, E. L. (2019). Mentoring students engaging in scholarly projects and dissertations in doctoral nursing programs. *Nursing Outlook, 67*(6), 776–788. https://doi.org/10.1016/j.outlook.2019.06.021

Cleary, M., Thapa, D. K., West, S., Lopez, V., Williamson, M., Sahay, A., & Kornhaber, R. (2023). Mentoring students in doctoral nursing programs: A scoping review. *Journal of Professional Nursing: Official Journal of the American Association of Colleges of Nursing, 45*, 71–88. https://doi.org/10.1016/j.profnurs.2023.01.010

Dunlap, J. J., Brewer, T. L., & Mainous, R. O. (2023). External scholarship mentors for DNP-prepared faculty: A practice-oriented exemplar. *Nurse Educator, 48*(5), 240–246. https://doi.org/10.1097/NNE.0000000000001409

Hardimann, M. (2012). *The brain targeted teaching model for 21st-century schools*. Corwin.

Milner, K. A., Hays, D., Farus-Brown, S., Zonsius, M. C., & Fineout-Overholt, E. (2023). National evaluation of DNP projects based on 2015 AACN white paper and 2019 DNP project roadmap. *Journal of Professional Nursing: Official Journal of the American Association of Colleges of Nursing, 48*, 60–65. https://doi.org/10.1016/j.profnurs.2023.05.002

Mitchell, K. M., McMillan, D. E., Lobchuk, M.M., Nickel, N.C., Rabbani, R., & Li, J. (2021). Development and validation of the Situated Academic

Writing Self-Efficacy Scale (SAWSES). *Assessing Writing, 48*(2021), 100524. https://doi.org/10.1016/j.aws.2021.100524

Smeltzer, S. C., Sharts-Hopko, N. C., Cantrell, M. A., Heverly, M. A., Wise, N. J., Jenkinson, A., & Nthenge, S. (2014). Challenges to research productivity of doctoral program nursing faculty. *Nursing Outlook, 62*(4), 268–274. https://doi.org/10.1016/j.outlook.2014.04.007

Sword, H., Trofimova, E. & Ballard, M. (2018). Frustrated academic writers. *Higher Education Research & Development, 37*(4), 852–867.

# Pathways to Successful Academic Writing for Doctor of Nursing Practice Projects

## Objectives

- Interpret academic writing within the discipline of nursing.
- Explore strategies to build emotional fitness for academic writing and publishing.
- Discover resources for writing self-assessment.
- Develop an academic writing improvement plan.

### Opening Scenario

Dr. Duran began her discussion by stating, "As you moved through your graduate program, you followed assignment guidelines and were evaluated using rubrics to help you develop your writing skills. The more you practiced, the more proficient you became. Academic writing and publishing are very similar. You will start as a beginner, and then practice skills that help you publish your work. You already have part of the content knowledge you need, because your experience as a clinician provides insight into what is important and relevant to your population."

Dr. Avila replied, "Knowing that helps me feel a little less lost! There's so much that is new but understanding that I can connect even a small part of it to what I already know is so helpful." Dr. Duran continues, "I'll try to help you do that as we progress through each step of the process. Some of the first steps will include investigating what academic writing means in nursing and the importance of connecting your work to what has already been published. You'll also need to be aware of how important it is to be an emotionally fit writer. Emotional fitness means taking frustrations and setbacks in stride and considering them part of the process. In the clinical setting, you are well acquainted with the kind of normal frustrations that arise daily, and they don't cause you to quit your job. Sometimes, though, we let the normal frustrations of writing completely derail a project and cause us to quit. Once you understand that writing can be a highly emotional process, you'll understand how important it will be to build your emotional fitness level so that you can view the frustrations as part of the process. Fortunately, there are excellent resources available to familiarize you with academic writing in the nursing discipline, assess your emotional fitness, and assist with developing a self-improvement plan."

## Defining Academic Writing Within the Discipline of Nursing

If you were asked what your favorite genre of movies is, you'd probably be able to answer without hesitation. Crime dramas, romantic comedies, or science fiction, perhaps? But when it comes to genres of writing, most of us are often unsure of what that means. *Genre* comes from the French meaning "kind or sort" and refers to a category of artistic, musical, or literary composition characterized by a particular style, form, or content (Merriam-Webster, n.d.).

Therefore, we can view academic writing as a category of literary composition. The form, style, and content are driven by the discipline of the writer and target audience, which means each discipline has its specialized language and evidence base. For example, writing for practicing nurses is usually very different than writing for researchers or theorists. And within each discipline, every journal has its focus, target audience, and style of writing. No wonder it's so easy to get confused!

Here is a helpful definition of academic writing for nursing:

> specialized in nursing, communicates original thought, includes support from the literature, contains formal language consistent with the discipline, and is formatted in a manner consistent with peer-reviewed publications. (Hunker et al., 2014, p. 1)

It can be helpful to examine that definition in detail, especially the first two items: "specialized in nursing" and "inclusive of original thoughts." Both can easily create confusion about the actual meaning, so we'll spend some time on the definitions we are using in this book.

## Specializing in Nursing (Nursing's Disciplinary Perspective or Focus)

Hunker et al. (2014) use the idea of "specialized in nursing" to apply to academic writing. A broader definition is provided in "The Essentials: Core Competencies for Professional Nursing Education" (American Association of Colleges of Nursing, 2021). This definition states that demonstrating an understanding of nursing's distinct perspective is an important competency in all areas of the profession and does not limit the definition to writing. Unfortunately, identifying nursing's perspective is often neglected. Such professional neglect of our specialized perspective means nursing's unique contribution to health care can easily be lost. Consider the great loss to health care if the improvements toward advanced nursing care that arise from doctor of nursing practice (DNP) projects are not viewed through a "disciplinary lens" and therefore not identified as nursing.

An excellent way to highlight nursing's distinct focus is by using nursing theories during project development and implementation, and in reporting the results. Theories show how specific ideas (or concepts) are related (Roy, 2018). Eminent nursing scholars have made a collective plea for using unifying central concepts or theory to maintain nursing's disciplinary focus and provide support for building accumulated disciplinary knowledge (Fawcett, 2014,

2017; Newman et al., 2008; Reed, 2017; Roy, 2018; Thorne & Sawatzky, 2014).

If theory is used consistently in DNP project reports, authors can synthesize and build new connections and knowledge related to the theory. Think of the body of literature on a certain topic as an ongoing conversation with many people involved. Each article can be thought of as one person in the conversation, with all the articles making up a group discussion or conversation. Conversations are interactive, with those involved contributing ideas and original thoughts and making an effort to connect their ideas to the conversation in progress. If there is no interaction, and only one person speaks, it is a monologue instead of a conversation. A scholarly work that is not connected to the discipline through theory can easily become disconnected from what has already been published, and the work becomes more of a scholarly monologue than a scholarly conversation (Monsivais, 2019). Think of using theory as an excellent method of connecting your work to the larger scholarly conversation in the literature.

## Connecting to the Scholarly Conversation

Unfortunately, nurse authors do not often use theory to connect published DNP projects to the larger scholarly conversation. In a review of 191 DNP project reports, only 33% of the reviewed reports described a theoretical framework to guide the project (Turkson-Ocran et al., 2020). While it is impossible to know the reasons that so few of the published reports contained a theoretical framework, one recurring possibility may be that DNP authors aren't familiar with frameworks that are a good match to nurse practitioner practice. This section will provide an overview of models and theories that have applicability for nurse practitioner practice.

Levine's conservation model (Schaefer et al., 1991) is especially applicable to nurse practitioners. Odesina et al. (2010) carried out a quality improvement project using Levine's model to improve sickle cell pain management in an emergency department, providing a noteworthy example of the application of the model. And in an example of a broader application of the theory, Abumaria et al.

(2015) describe the adaptation of Levine's model as a framework for advanced gerontology nursing practice. Kolcaba's comfort theory (Kolcaba, 1994) is applicable to a wide range of practice settings, and has been studied extensively since it was first published. Krinsky et al. (2014) and Lafond et al. (2019) provide examples of applying the theory to practice.

A good strategy to identify helpful theories for your project is to review intervention implications for advanced practice nurses that emerge from research reports. For example, Joly (2015), Orr et al. (2020), and Zhao et al. (2020) use Meleis's transitions theory (Meleis et al., 2000) to examine the challenges in transitioning across health care services for specific groups of patients (young people with medically complex conditions, patients who have undergone a laryngectomy, and adolescent mothers of NICU patients being discharged to home, respectively). The numerous challenges for any given patient population are often within the scope of advanced practice nurses, who can use quality improvement measures to coordinate services and intervene at the system level to mitigate some of the challenges. If the interventions are then reported in the literature and tied back into the theory, the scholarly conversation about care transitions becomes more meaningful to those wanting to improve health care outcomes for patients experiencing care transitions.

Research stemming from Leininger's theory of culture care diversity and universality (McFarland & Wehbe-Alamah, 2019) offers other examples of potential interventions applicable to nurse practitioner practice. Chiatti (2019) found that language preference, dietary practice, and family dynamics played an integral role in the health and well-being of an immigrant population. The results of that study and many others provide advanced practice nurses with specific information that they can use to improve health outcomes. If the interventions are then reported in the literature and tied back to the theory, the scholarly conversation about cultural practices becomes more meaningful to those wanting to improve outcomes. An excellent resource for theory-guided practice examples can be found on the Nursology website (https://nursology.net).

In addition to nursing theories, classic change theories can be incorporated into the project. Classic change theories include organizational and behavioral theories of change and therefore cover a broader scope than nursing theory. Some well-known change theories are Lewin's Force Field Analysis, Lippitts's model of change, and Bandura's social cognitive theory. Nursing theories provide a focused framework to guide nursing practice and connect the practice to patient outcomes. When nursing theories and classic change theories are used together, they provide a more comprehensive approach to improving outcomes than using either one alone (White, 2021a).

As you develop a manuscript from your DNP project report, it's always helpful to see how other nurse authors incorporate nursing theory and change theories into their project reports. In addition to searching library databases for published articles, searching university-based DNP project repositories provides access to a large number of DNP project reports. Some examples of university-based DNP project repositories are the Johns Hopkins School of Nursing (n.d.), The University of Texas at El Paso College of Nursing (n.d.), and Vanderbilt University School of Nursing (n.d). Additionally, Doctors of Nursing Practice (Doctorsofnursingpractice.org) is an online resource that archives DNP projects from across the country on a fee basis.

## Making a Place for Your Work in the Literature

"Original thoughts" can be a confusing idea in academic writing, as the idea of what is original in academic writing may not be similar to the idea of originality when writing fiction or music. You may be surprised by what it means in academic writing. When you conduct a literature review and evaluate published evidence by assessing literature findings such as the strength of the studies, settings, or population, this represents *your* evaluation and therefore your original thoughts. Similarly, your identification of a knowledge gap in published literature also represents original thought.

In academic writing, showing you are "in charge" of the literature by evaluating it, building your argument about what should be done, and identifying new ideas from reviews of the literature all fall under the definition of original thoughts (Clark & Sousa, 2018, Kamler & Thomson, 2014). Information synthesis is the key to identifying those new ideas, and therefore an essential skill. Like many novice authors, you may be in the habit of "serial citing" (Monsivais & Robbins, 2020), but with practice, you will become more proficient at synthesizing rather than individually citing pieces of information from each article. Then don't forget that when you identify the nursing theory that best links your work to the scholarly conversation that is already in progress, that is also your original thought. In summary, your evaluation of the literature, identification of a knowledge gap in which to situate your work, and use of a particular theory are all ways that count as original thought in academic writing.

## DNP Project Reports: A Specialized Category of Academic Writing

Nursing's disciplinary focus, connecting to the scholarly conversation, and making a place for your work in the literature are not the only areas to consider as you develop your manuscript. The project design and reporting guidelines will also influence the development of your academic writing.

### Project Design

For DNP reports, the project design is typically based on evidence-based practice (EBP), quality improvement (QI), or a combination of both. The idea of EBP is certainly not new. The push for the EBP movement is credited to Dr. Archie Cochrane, who in the early 1970s criticized the lack of evidence summaries of randomized controlled trials on which to base practice (Cochrane, 1989). His visionary work laid the foundation for the Cochrane Collaboration, a global network dedicated to providing high-quality synthesized evidence for making healthcare decisions.

To make sure that we are all using the same definition of EBP, let's look at a widely accepted definition from the Agency for Healthcare Research and Quality (n.d.):

> A way of providing health care that is guided by a thoughtful integration of the best available scientific knowledge with clinical expertise. This approach allows the practitioner to critically assess research data, clinical guidelines, and other information resources to correctly identify the clinical problem, apply the most high-quality intervention, and re-evaluate the outcome for future improvement. (para. 1)

Models and frameworks representing EBP are numerous, and the choices can seem overwhelming at first glance. Fortunately, there are commonalities among the models, making it a little easier to find out which might be the best match for your project. The commonalities include problem identification, searching for the best evidence, evaluating the evidence, recommending for or against change, implementing change if recommended, and evaluating outcomes of the implementation (White, 2021b). Two popular models being used to guide evidence into practice include the Johns Hopkins Nursing EBP model and guidelines (Dang et al., 2022) and the advancing research and clinical practice through close collaboration model (Melnyk et al., 2021).

In addition to EBP models, quality improvement models are often used in DNP project design. A widely accepted definition comes from the Centers for Medicare and Medicaid Services (2021):

> Quality improvement is the framework used to systematically improve care. Quality improvement seeks to standardize processes and structures to reduce variation, achieve predictable results, and improve outcomes for patients, healthcare systems, and organizations. Structure includes things like technology, culture, leadership, and physical capital; process includes knowledge capital (e.g., standard operating procedures) or human capital (e.g., education and training). (para. 2)

A key point to bear in mind is that quality improvement projects are often focused or based on local data that is specific to one institution. The results are therefore limited to a particular setting or population. Examples of this type of project include reducing medication error rates or improving the use of infection prevention measures to decrease catheter-associated urinary tract infections.

More recently, implementation science has been recognized as an important component of the process in EBP and/or QI. Implementation science is frequently defined using one of the earliest definitions cited in the literature as "the scientific study of methods to promote the systematic uptake of research findings and other evidence-based practices into routine practice, and, hence, to improve the quality and effectiveness of health services" (Eccles & Mittman, 2006, p. 1).

Implementation science provides a key link between best practice and the best way to implement that practice. Implementation can be influenced at multiple levels of any healthcare system. For example, patient, provider, organization, and policy levels may individually or in combination influence the implementation process (Bauer et al., 2015). Studying factors that influence implementation falls under the broad purview of implementation science, as does identifying institution-specific approaches for bringing the best evidence into practice. With a focus on nursing, Roberts et al. (2023) detail the value of integrating implementation science into practice and research.

In summary, DNP project designs frequently include EBP, QI, and implementation science methods or a combination of them. These frameworks guide the process of bringing new knowledge into practice. When partnered with a change theory (to consider an organizational or behavioral change) and nursing theory (to consider disciplinary practice), published DNP projects provide a comprehensive guide to improving advanced nursing practice.

## Reporting Guidelines

Standardized reporting guidelines allow for comparison of quality improvement projects published in the literature. The ability to compare designs, implementation strategies, and outcomes allows practitioners to choose the best evidence for their practice. The

Enhancing the Quality and Transparency of Health Research Network (www.equator-network.org/) provides a large number of reporting guidelines, among them the QI reporting guideline known as SQUIRE2.0 (Standards for Quality Improvement Reporting Excellence). Standardized reporting guidelines are another strategy for adding your work to the larger scholarly conversation, as their use makes it easier for others to compare your design, implementation, and outcomes to those who have published before you.

# Emotional Fitness for Academic Writing and Publishing

If you have always thought of writing as simply formatting, sentence structure, grammar, and other mechanics related to creating a document, it might surprise you to find out how much more might be involved. Have you considered that writing is an emotionally charged activity? Knowing what your own emotions are about academic writing is an essential starting point. Many new authors have never given much thought to the role that emotions play in successful academic writing. But without that knowledge, you're likely to decide to set aside your writing project when it isn't going well. Take a few minutes to think about what excites you and what scares you about academic writing. There's no right or wrong answer, and each person's answer will be based on their own prior experiences.

## Collage Exercise

The following collage exercise is a thought-provoking way for you to gain insight into your emotions about academic writing and publishing. For this exercise, you'll need some magazines or other print media that can be cut up or torn. You'll also need a poster board or paper that is approximately 2.0 x 2.5 feet. Larger is fine, but not necessary. While the exercise can be carried out individually, sharing the meaning of the pictures and words with colleagues creates a more meaningful experience.

Start by dividing your poster board into four equal sections with labels as shown.

| Section 1. Sitting down to write your manuscript | Section 3. Receiving feedback about the manuscript |
| --- | --- |
| Section 2. Submitting your manuscript to the journal | Section 4. Seeing your article in print |

Once the board is labeled, look through the magazines for pictures or words that reflect your thoughts and feelings about each of the sections. Cut or tear them out of the magazine, and glue them in the appropriate section. For section 1, you'll look for pictures or words that reflect your feelings about sitting down to write a manuscript that you will submit for publication. For section 2, you'll look for words or pictures that reflect your feelings about submitting the manuscript for publication. For section 3, you'll look for words or pictures that reflect how you feel about receiving feedback that major revisions are needed, or the manuscript has been rejected. For section 4, you'll look for words and pictures that reflect your thoughts and feelings about seeing your work in print.

Once you have finished cutting out the pictures, if you are doing the exercise with a group of colleagues, share the meaning of the words and pictures in each section. The collage exercise should convince you that writing has a strong emotional component, and unfortunately it's often negative. Recent workshop participants shared their responses to the collage exercise, demonstrating an incredibly wide range of emotions. When it came to sitting down to write, the responses included dread, being an explorer who is lost, feeling like an imposter, feeling vulnerable, difficulty engaging my brain with the task, not knowing where to start, and wondering if ideas are publication-worthy. Responses to emotions related to sending it out included feelings of relief, some mixed emotions about whether it was the right journal to submit to, anxiety, nervousness, and being unworthy. Receiving the review brought up feelings of being excited, scared, and helpful, as well as feelings of pain, anger, and grief. Seeing one's work in print generally brings up positive emotions such as being fulfilled, proud, and feeling validated that peers thought the manuscript was worthy of publishing. For some, however, the imposter syndrome persists after publication now that the work is available to a larger audience.

There's a good reason for using a paper collage instead of a digital format. The creative process can often flourish more easily in a paper-based environment. That's because digital pictures pasted on an electronic document may remind you of work and lecture development, which might initiate stress and therefore can suppress free thought and creativity (Martindale & Greenough, 1973). Additionally, searching for pictures through a search engine requires an individual to know how they feel before having a chance to explore a variety of pictures. Often, seeing a picture while turning magazine pages can induce an emotion that has been unrecognized until seeing the picture.

Creativity involves bringing new ideas to light and engages multiple processes in the brain (Jung & Vartanian, 2018). Finding pictures and creating collages to explain abstract thoughts has the potential to bring forward emotions that may have been buried under thoughts about work and responsibility. Developing collages is a creative process, as the content is novel (your thoughts and your pictures) and has the utility to help us grow by bringing forward emotions and issues (Runco & Jaeger, 2012) that we may not have thought about related to publishing. So, although a paper collage can be viewed as old-fashioned and old-school, the creative process is enhanced when it is used.

Regardless of your ability to structure sentences or use correct grammar, remember that negative emotions can get in the way of writing. Developing emotional fitness for the process will allow you to take the frustrations and negativity in stride and see them as a normal part of the process. Taking some time to reflect on your current level of emotional fitness for writing is time well spent and provides insight into what you may need to do to improve your writing fitness level. We'll talk about some of the ways to build writing emotional fitness in next.

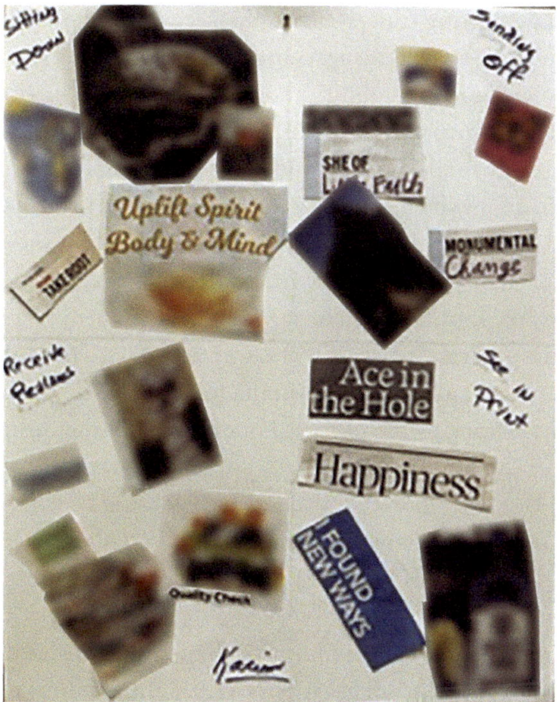


**FIGURE 2.1**  Collage exercise example from one of the workshop participants.

## Understanding That Frustration Is Part of the Process

Undoubtedly, you've built emotional fitness for your faculty role. Frustrations come along regularly and may include situations in which students make seemingly unreasonable requests, or policies that are puzzling but must be followed. But you know those types of situations are just part of the job because you've experienced them before and have learned how to cope with them. Certainly, the routine frustrations in academia would not cause you to resign from your job. Similarly, academic writing comes with its own set of normal frustrations and should not be seen as a sign that you should abandon the project. Frustrations may include difficulties scheduling writing time, writer's block, requested revisions that you don't agree with, disagreements with coauthors, and constant feelings of vulnerability about the process. Then, of course, there's the disheartening experience of having your manuscript rejected after spending time and energy making requested revisions. No doubt you have your personalized list of the frustrations of writing!

Rather than allowing those frustrations to interfere with your progress, try reframing them so you can view them as a normal part of the process. Sword (2017) suggests picking a metaphor that appeals to you and using it to put the frustrations that come with academic writing in perspective. For example, gardening includes a range of expected activities such as planting, watering, and fertilizing. But then there are also less pleasant ones such as plants that die or weeds that overtake the garden. Gardeners accept those frustrations as part of gardening, and don't consider them a reason to quit gardening.

How about traveling? Planning to go somewhere you haven't been before for a conference or vacation is exciting, and we always anticipate the trip will go according to our plans. That's a rarity. Flight delays or cancellations can derail the most careful planning, but you know that is a normal occurrence. You're willing to persevere to get to the end goal of your final destination because you think the goal is important. Similarly, your goals with academic writing will help you keep moving forward if you accept frustrations as a normal part of the process.

## Becoming the Writer You Want to Be

If you've identified your emotions related to academic writing and developed an understanding that frustrations are a normal part of the process, you're off to a great start in creating a growth mind-set about academic writing. A growth mind-set encompasses the idea that you can develop needed writing habits and skills and use them to improve your writing. Developing expertise in any skill demands choosing experiences and activities that help you develop that skill. Writing fitness is no different. Important activities that will help you develop as a writer include prioritizing writing times by scheduling them, participating in professional development opportunities, and committing to behaviors that support physical and emotional health and wellness.

When you prioritize writing time by scheduling it on your calendar, you show your commitment to developing your writing fitness. Try and capitalize on times when you can concentrate the best. For some of us that's first thing in the morning, and for others late at night. Aim for times when you won't be interrupted. More frequent sessions for shorter periods are generally more productive. While it is natural to think that you'll need to schedule large blocks of time (like a whole day) to accomplish anything, the reality is that productivity declines for most people after about 3 hours, so if you can block 3 hours, great! But if 30 minutes a day is your reality, then try that. And writing time may not always be the literal act of writing. Since reading is a vital part of academic writing, when you spend time reading background articles, that may be your "writing" time for that day. And a space designated for writing is important, whether it's a whole office or a corner of your kitchen table. That space sends a signal to your brain that says, "It's time to write!"

Many universities provide professional development opportunities in academic writing, so take advantage of them. It's also a great way to meet faculty from outside your discipline and learn what they are doing. Writing partnerships often develop at these types of sessions.

In addition to scheduling writing time and professional development, your commitment to behaviors that support physical and emotional health and wellness is vitally important. Proper nutrition, exercise, and restorative rest contribute greatly to being an effective writer who has the emotional fitness to deal with the uncertainties inherent in writing and publishing. Creativity and new ideas flourish in a rested brain!

Sword (2017) categorizes the foundational habits of successful writers into what she calls "BASE" habits. The acronym stands for behavioral (making time and space for writing), artisanal (ongoing skill development), social (interaction and feedback with others), and emotional (thinking that emphasizes pleasure and growth).

## Assess Yourself

Use the Writer's Diet free online tool (www.writersdiet.com/base) to help identify your strengths and weaknesses in behavioral, artisanal, social, and emotional habits. You'll also find suggestions to strengthen your habits. What did you find out about yourself and scholarly writing when you looked at your results? Did you find (like many others) that frustration and anxiety were at the top of your list? Were you intrigued to find out more about how to make writing less frustrating and anxiety producing?

We took Sword's BASE assessment and here's what we found out: Diane and Fran demonstrate positive emotions toward writing, but they tend to write in isolation and therefore could benefit from improving their social habits. In contrast, Leslie demonstrates good social habits but would benefit from strengthening behavioral habits. Our collective writing habits are continually being strengthened by the chance to create collaborative work!

### Case Study of Novice Faculty Member Designing an Improvement Plan

As a new faculty member, Dr. Avila is new to both teaching and scholarly publishing. Dr. Duran looks encouragingly at Dr. Avila and says, "I'm glad to see that you took the BASE assessment and then made an overall plan for yourself. I know you were interested in looking for workshops to attend and were also trying to figure out how to collaborate more with colleagues. What we can do in this session is figure out exactly how you can do those, so let me know what you've been thinking about since you took the assessment. Dr. Avila sighs deeply and says, "It feels overwhelming because I look at my schedule each day, and there's so much in every day and I feel like so much of it's out of my control. I'm just not even sure how to take control of the time so that I can make these plans work. Do you have any ideas?"

Dr. Duran smiles knowingly. "That's a very common problem for a lot of people, and I can give you a few tips that I've seen work for others and me. Let's talk about writing time first. It should be scheduled just like everything else you do that is important, so it should show up on your calendar as protected time and should be honored just as your other work commitments are. The time that you pick to schedule this writing time ideally is based on the time you are best able to concentrate and focus. When would that be for you? Dr. Avila says, "I think afternoons would work for me because I teach in the morning usually, so by afternoon things settle down a bit and I could focus on my writing. Most weeks, Monday, Tuesday, and Thursday afternoons would work." Dr. Duran advises her to schedule 1 hour on each of those days to dedicate to writing and to make sure she is in a place where she won't be interrupted. "Sometimes people will put a note outside their office door that they're in a conference, or they work in another area like the library or at home." Dr. Avila says, "That sounds very doable, and I think for me it would work best in my office. If I put a note outside that said I was busy, I think my colleagues will honor that because they know I'm new and that I'm trying to get started in this writing area."

Dr. Duran continues, "Your commitment to 3 hours a week of dedicated time for your scholarship is an important step toward your success in academia. And remember, although we call it 'writing time,' everything you do toward creating your final manuscript is part of that time. Reading, thinking, or finding articles all support your final goal, and you'll find that you will be able to make excellent progress by dedicating 3 hours per week. You've also said that you're interested in attending workshops about writing. Were you able to find any?" Dr. Avila informs her that she has identified a couple of upcoming workshops within driving distance and another that is an online workshop 1 hour a week for 5 weeks and that provides feedback on writing. She says she'd like to try both the in-person and online workshops, but the online one was kind of expensive. Dr. Duran agrees that both would be good learning experiences and offers to investigate funding that might support the online workshop.

"Now that you have identified some professional development opportunities, let's talk about how you might build collaboration with colleagues for writing," said Dr. Duran. Have you thought about two or three colleagues who might be willing to work with you on writing? Dr. Avila looks perplexed and says, "That's a hard question, and this is the part I'm struggling with the most because, being new on the faculty here, I don't have any real close friends yet. Frankly, I'm scared to ask people to critique my work because what if they think I'm stupid, and what if they wonder how I was even hired?" Dr. Duran nods understandingly. "I want to reassure you that your fears are common, but most of our faculty will think highly of you for being proactive about advancing your scholarship. Most of us remember all too well what it feels like to be a novice faculty member. We do have a few faculty who are newer to their positions and who have also just come out of DNP programs within the last few years and would be great collaborators with you. If you would be interested in forming a writing group, I would be glad to facilitate it, as I know you all have a common interest in publishing. You've made excellent progress in putting your plan to advance your scholarship in place, and I think the results will be worth the effort."

## Demonstrating the Collage Exercise

Dr. Duran meets with Dr. Avila after she has completed the collage exercise and asks "Can you tell me about those pictures that demonstrated how you felt about sitting down to write? Dr. Avila responds with emotion, "The angry ocean scene is kind of how I felt when I sit down to write because it brings back the feelings of when I got some very negative feedback in my doctoral program. I was told they were not sure I was ever going to be a good writer, so when I think about that, my stomach churns kind of like that ocean

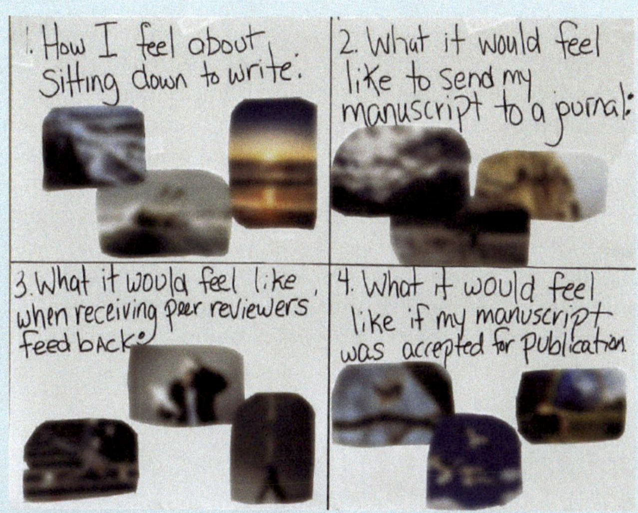


**FIGURE 2.2** Collage exercise.

churns. But then I also have the sunrise because I had some other faculty along the way in my DNP who encouraged me to develop an article for publication. They told me my project was a strong one and that it was well written. That for me was the opposite of a stomach-churning experience and more of a wonderful beginning like a sunrise. But overall I guess when I sit down I still have some anxiety and some real nervousness about my ability to be a good writer, and I know that I need to do something about my negative self-talk."

Dr. Duran reassures her that those feelings are normal and part of the growth process for new faculty. She then asks about the pictures reflecting what it would feel like to send a manuscript off for peer review. Dr. Avila brings up a vivid metaphor: "It's kind of like the swinging bridge because I want to cross to the other side, and I know it's a safe walk, but it will feel a little bit scary as the wind blows the bridge a bit and I might be thrown slightly off balance. But I reach for the guard rails to steady myself and keep walking slowly. I think that my metaphorical guardrails are my mentors and colleagues." Dr. Duran then asks her to describe the next set of pictures about her perception of what receiving a peer review on her manuscript would be like. Dr. Avila continues, "I've heard colleagues talk about receiving scathing reviews from journals. I would be scared the same thing will happen to me, and that I'd completely lose my confidence. I think I would feel totally crushed and flattened and not want to continue with further submissions." Dr. Duran moves to the next set of pictures, which are birds in flight and a rainbow, and Dr. Avila explains she chose them because if she had an article in print, she would feel like she was soaring because she had accomplished her hard-won goal of being a writer with the pot-of-gold rainbow at the other end.

## Your Turn!

Now that you have done your self-assessment of writing, what kind of behavioral, artisanal, social, and emotional goals do you have for yourself? What are some strategies you have identified to help you achieve those goals?

# Chapter Wrap-Up

| Knowledge | Skills | Resources |
|---|---|---|
| Academic writing in the discipline of nursing | Apply middle-range nursing-focused theories to clinical situations.<br><br>Situate your work in the literature by evaluating what has already been done and establishing the need for your work. | Fawcett, J. (2017)<br><br>Clark, A., & Sousa, B. (2018) |
| Project design, quality improvement, evidence-based practice, and implementation science | Apply EBP or QI frameworks.<br><br>Become familiar with implementation science concepts. | Dang et al. (2022)<br><br>Roberts et al. (2023) |

| Knowledge | Skills | Resources |
|---|---|---|
| Change theories | Apply a change theory to your project. | White (2021a) |
| Reporting guidelines | Use appropriate reporting guidelines. | Enhancing the Quality and Transparency of Health Research (EQUATOR) network. SQUIRE (QI) and SQUIRE.edu |
| Importance of emotional fitness | Identify own strengths/challenges. Reframe frustration. Prioritize wellness practices. Develop social and emotional habits that support writing. Develop an improvement plan. | Collage exercise<br><br>Texts or articles or assessments (www.writersdiet.com/base) |

# References


Abumaria, I. M., Hastings-Tolsma, M., & Sakraida, T. J. (2015). Levine's conservation model: A framework for advanced gerontology nursing practice. *Nursing Forum, 50*(3), 179–188. https://doi.org/10.1111/nuf.12077

Agency for Healthcare Research and Quality (n.d.). Topic: Evidence-based practice. https://www.ahrq.goopics/evidence-based-practice.html

American Association of Colleges of Nursing. (2021). The Essentials: Core competencies for professional nursing education. Accessible online at ihttps://www.aacnnursing.org/Portals/0/PDFs/Publications/Essentials-2021.pdf

Bauer, M. S., Damschroder, L., Hagedorn, H., Smith, J., & Kilbourne, A. M. (2015). An introduction to implementation science for the non-specialist. *BMC Psychology, 3*(1), 32. https://doi.org/10.1186/s40359-015-0089-9

Centers for Medicare and Medicaid Services. (2021). *Quality measurement and quality improvement.* https://www.cms.gov/Medicare/Quality-Initiatives-Patient-Assessment-Instruments/MMS/Quality-Measure-and-Quality-Improvement-

Chiatti, B. D. (2019). Culture care beliefs and practices of Ethiopian immigrants. *Journal of Transcultural Nursing: Official Journal of the Transcultural Nursing Society, 30*(4), 340–349. https://doi.org/10.1177/1043659618817589

Clark, A., & Sousa, B. (2018). *How to be a happy academic*. SAGE.

Cochrane, A. L. (1989). Archie Cochrane in his own words. Selections arranged from his 1972 introduction to "Effectiveness and efficiency: Random reflections on the health services" 1972. *Controlled Clinical Trials, 10*(4), 428–433. https://doi.org/10.1016/0197-2456(89)90008-1

Dang, D., Dearholt, S., Bissett, K., Ascenzi, J., & Whalen, M. (2022). *Johns Hopkins evidence-based practice for nurses and healthcare professionals: Model and guidelines* (4th ed.). Sigma Theta Tau International.

Eccles, M. P., & Mittman, B. S. (2006). Welcome to implementation science. *Implementation Science, 1*(1), 1–3. https://doi.org/10.1186/1748-5908-1-1

Fawcett, J. (2014). Thoughts about conceptual models, theories, and quality improvement projects. *Nursing Science Quarterly, 27*(4), 336–339.

Fawcett, J. (2017). *Applying conceptual models of nursing. Quality improvement, research, and practice*. Springer.

Hunker, D. F., Gazza, E. A., & Shellenbarger, T. (2014). Evidence-based knowledge, skills, and attitudes for scholarly writing development across all levels of nursing education. *Journal of Professional Nursing: Official Journal of the American Association of Colleges of Nursing, 30*(4), 341–346. https://doi.org/10.1016/j.profnurs.2013.11.003

Johns Hopkins University School of Nursing (n.d.). *DNP final project*. https://nursing.jhu.edu/programs/doctoral/dnp/capstone/

Joly, E. (2015). Transition to adulthood for young people with medical complexity: An integrative literature review. *Journal of Pediatric Nursing, 30*(5), 91. S0882–5963(15)00189-X

Jung, R. E., & Vartanian, O. (Eds.) (2018). *The Cambridge handbook of the neuroscience of creativity*. Cambridge University Press.

Kamler, B., & Thomson, P. (2014) *Helping doctoral students write. Pedagogies for supervision*. Routledge.

Kolcaba, K. (1994). A theory of comfort for nursing. *Journal of Advanced Nursing, 19*, 1178–184.

Krinsky, R., Murillo, I., & Johnson, J. (2014). A practical application of Katharine Kolcaba's comfort theory to cardiac patients. *Applied Nursing Research, 27*(2), 147–150. https://doi.org/10.1016/j.apnr.2014.02.004

Lafond, D. A., Bowling, S., Fortkiewicz, J. M., Reggio, C., & Hinds, P. S. (2019). Integrating the comfort theory™ into pediatric primary palliative care to improve access to care. *Journal of Hospice and Palliative Nursing: The Official Journal of the Hospice and Palliative Nurses Association, 21*(5), 382–389. https://doi.org/10.1097/NJH.0000000000000538

Martindale, C., & Greenough, J. (1973). The differential effect of increased arousal on creative and intellectual performance. *Journal of Genetic Psychology, 123,* 329–335.

McFarland, M. R., & Wehbe-Alamah, H. B. (2019). Leininger's theory of culture care diversity and universality: An overview with a historical retrospective and a view toward the future. *Journal of Transcultural Nursing: Official Journal of the Transcultural Nursing Society, 30*(6), 540–557. https://doi.org/10.1177/1043659619867134

Meleis, A. I., Sawyer, L. M., Im, E. O., Hilfinger Messias, D. K., & Schumacher, K. (2000). Experiencing transitions: An emerging middle-range theory. *Advances in Nursing Science, 23*(1), 12–28. https://doi.org/10.1097/00012272-200009000-00006

Melnyk, B. M., Tan, A., Hsieh, A. P., & Gallagher-Ford, L. (2021). Evidence-based practice culture and mentorship predict EBP implementation, nurse job satisfaction, and intent to stay: Support for the ARCC© model. *Worldviews on Evidence-Based Nursing, 18*(4), 272–281. https://doi.org/10.1111/wvn.12524

Merriam-Webster. (n.d.). *Genre.* https://www.merriam-webster.com/dictionary/genre

Monsivais, D. B. (2019). Scholarly monologues or scholarly conversations? Theory can make the difference. *Research and Theory for Nursing Practice, 33*(2), 113–114.

Monsivais, D. B., & Robbins, L. K. (2020). Don't be a serial citer. Synthesize! *Nursing Education Perspectives, 41*(1), 65–66. https://doi.org/10.1097/01.NEP.0000000000000419

Newman, M. A., Smith, M. C., Pharris, M. D., & Jones, D. (2008). The focus of the discipline revisited. *Advances in Nursing Science, 1*(31), E16–E27.

Odesina, V., Bellini, S, Delaney, C., Bacarro, N., Lundquist, K., D'Angelo, S. Goodrich, S. (2010). Evidence-based sickle cell pain management in the emergency department. *Advanced Emergency Nursing Journal, 32*(2), 102–111.

Orr, E., Ballantyne, M., Gonzalez, A., & Jack, S. M. (2020). The complexity of the NICU-to-home experience for adolescent mothers: Meleis' transitions theory applied. *Advances in Nursing Science, 43*(4), 349–359. https://doi.org/10.1097/ANS.0000000000000299

Reed, P. G. (2017). Philosophical clarity and justifying the scope of advanced practice nursing. *Nursing Science Quarterly, 30*(1), 73–76.

Roberts, N. A., Young, A. M., & Duff, J. (2023). Using implementation science in nursing research. *Seminars in Oncology Nursing, 39*(2), 151399. https://doi.org/10.1016/j.soncn.2023.151399

Roy, C. (2018). Nursing knowledge in the 21st century. Domain-derived and basic science practice-shaped. *Advances in Nursing Science, 42*(1), 28–42.

Runco, M., & Jaeger, G. J. (2012). The standard definition of creativity. *Creativity Research Journal, 21*, 92–96.

Schaefer, K. M., Pond, J. B., Levine, M. E., & Fawcett, F. (1991). *Levine's conservation model: A framework for nursing practice.* F.A. Davis Co.

Sword, H. (2017). *Air & light & time & space. How successful academics write.* Harvard University Press.

Thorne, S., & Sawatzky, R. (2014). Particularizing the general: Sustaining theoretical integrity in the context of an evidence-based practice agenda. *Advances in Nursing Science, 37*(1), 5–18. https://doi.org/10.1097/ANS.0000000000000011

Turkson-Ocran, R. N., Spaulding, E. M., Renda, S., Pandian, V., Rittler, H., Davidson, P. M., Nolan, M. T., & D'Aoust, R. (2020). A 10-year evaluation of projects in a doctor of nursing practice programme. *Journal of Clinical Nursing, 29*(21–22), 4090–4103. https://doi.org/10.1111/jocn.15435

The University of Texas at El Paso College of Nursing. (n.d.). *DNP scholarly project.* https://scholarworks.utep.edu/dnp_project/

Vanderbilt University School of Nursing. (n.d.). *DNP projects.* https://nursing.vanderbilt.edu/dnp/scholarlyproject.php

White, K. M. (2021a). Change theories and models: Framework for translation. In K. M. White, D. Dudley-Brown, & M. F. Terhaar (Eds.), *Translation of evidence into nursing and healthcare* (3rd ed., pp. 59–73). Springer.

White, K. M. (2021b). Evidence-based practice. In K. M. White, D. Dudley-Brown, & M.F. Terhaar (Eds.), *Translation of evidence into nursing and healthcare* (3rd ed., pp. 3–25). Springer.

# CHAPTER 3

# Coauthorship

Proceed With Caution!

## Objectives

- Define the benefits and challenges of coauthorship.
- Identify ethical concerns related to power differences between coauthors.
- Explore your motivation for academic writing.
- Familiarize yourself with resources for creating successful coauthorship collaborations.

### Opening Scenario

Dr. Avila approached Dr. Duran and hesitantly said, "Would it be possible for you to help me publish my DNP project? I want to learn how to publish so I can build my scholarship. Right before graduating, we were encouraged to seek a mentor to help us publish. I know you have published extensively, and I'd very much appreciate your guidance."

Dr. Duran says, "I'm glad to hear you recognize the importance of publishing your DNP project, and I'd be glad to guide you in the process. I'm getting a small group of DNP faculty together who are interested in publishing their DNP projects. We'll meet monthly, and I'll guide participants through the process. Writing projects are challenging, and the challenges are increased when there is a power difference between coauthors such as junior and senior faculty members or students and faculty members. Starting a writing project with clear expectations and written agreements is a best practice that will serve you well for the rest of your career. In the future, you may want to be able to guide your DNP students to publication, which means you need a solid grounding in the guidelines and need to know the resources available to help keep problems from developing. I'll go over some broad resources that will help you understand the most widely accepted definition of *authorship*, discuss why coauthorship needs very careful planning, and share resources with you to help you plan successful partnerships and coauthorship experiences. Partnership agreements may include a coauthorship role but do not have to. A partner may be someone who keeps you on track with your writing deadlines or who has agreed to provide constructive feedback on your work. You'll find that these types of agreements will be very useful tools that help minimize conflict as you work with colleagues."

## Defining Authorship

All too often, aspiring academic authors haven't read and understood the "gold standard" definition of *authorship*, which is foundational knowledge for any academic writing project. The widely accepted authorship definition comes from the International Committee of Medical Journal Editors (2024). The committee recommends the following four criteria be used to establish authorship (the list is taken from the Recommendations for the Conduct, Reporting, Editing, and Publication of Scholarly Work in Medical Journals):

1. Substantial contributions to the conception or design of the work; or the acquisition, analysis, or interpretation of data for the work; AND

2. Drafting the work or reviewing it critically for important intellectual content; AND

3. Final approval of the version to be published; AND

4. Agreement to be accountable for all aspects of the work in ensuring that questions related to the accuracy or integrity of any part of the work are appropriately investigated and resolved. In addition to being accountable for the parts of the work he or she has done, an author should be able to identify which co-authors are responsible for specific other parts of the work. In addition, authors should have confidence in the integrity of the contributions of their coauthors. All those designated as authors should meet all four criteria for authorship, and all who meet the four criteria should be identified as authors. (p.2)

The connections established by the "AND" at the end of each phrase are worth emphasizing. All four of those criteria should be present to establish authorship. In cases where all four of the criteria are not present, authorship credit should not be given. Instead, acknowledging specific contributions is appropriate.

The concept of authorship quickly increases in complexity when more than one author is involved. Unfortunately, formal guidelines related to coauthorship have not been established by national professional organizations. A national survey of 194 nursing faculty showed great variability in what criteria faculty used to determine coauthorship eligibility, highlighting the need for formal guidelines (Eiswirth & Fry, 2023). Becoming familiar with the potential complexities is well worth your time, as there are numerous benefits to coauthoring manuscripts. The following sections will acquaint you with the benefits and challenges of coauthorship and start you on the way to successful coauthor collaborations.

## Benefits of Coauthorship

Frequently, two or more authors decide to collaborate on a writing project and become coauthors. Coauthorship provides the chance to increase collaboration, exchange ideas (which may improve the quality of the manuscript), expand networks, mentor junior faculty in the publication process, and advance scholarship for the individuals involved and for the profession (Eiswirth & Fry, 2022; Oddi & Oddi, 2000). Coauthorship can result in undeniable benefits for the authors, including increasing the number of publications one may be able to write as an individual. Increased publication productivity often plays an important role in career advancement since publications are linked to promotion and tenure. Publications also are linked to increased professional visibility, which can widen career opportunities.

## Coauthorship Challenges

While coauthorship can be highly beneficial for those involved, it can also bring a wide array of challenges that make coauthorship a much more complex, lengthier, and chaotic process than single authorship (Eiswirth & Fry, 2022). Even the definition of *authorship* can be a point (or many points) of disgruntled discussion, as the International Committee of Medical Journal Editors provides only very broad guidelines that may be interpreted very differently by collaborating authors. For example, how much of a contribution is considered a "substantial" contribution? Is it drafting a certain percentage of the paper, and, if so, how much? Does a deep discussion when an idea is born and the project is designed qualify as authorship? And "reviewing it critically" covers a broad range of activities. It may mean providing feedback about the structure and flow of the writing, determining if the data analysis is valid, or if the data supports the conclusions.

Many of the complexities of coauthorship can be related to disciplinary norms related to manuscript development. Norms related to which sections, and how many sections, of the study each author should write based on their roles is an area that can differ markedly among disciplines. An understanding of what constitutes intellectual contribution is another area that differs. Being part of the research team and contributing to discussions may be considered an intellectual contribution worthy of authorship in some disciplines, leading to potential conflict (Smith & Master, 2017). In addition to the norms of each discipline, authors have their work styles and commitments. Some meet established deadlines, while others take a deadline as simply a suggestion. Each author on the team undoubtedly has specific professional or personal commitments that may impact their ability to meet deadlines for written drafts. What will happen when an author does not fulfill their commitment?

## Power Imbalances Create Additional Challenges

The challenges of coauthorship compound dramatically when there is a power differential between authors, as is the case with a junior and senior faculty member or a student–faculty authorship team. These raise ethical concerns, primarily related to the power differential of those working together. Nishikawa et al. (2015) provide a concise and comprehensive overview of the ethical concerns related to coauthorship. Junior faculty or students may be reluctant to state ideas or ask questions if they think there will be negative consequences for them. For example, if those with more power take undeserved credit for authorship, it can lead to insufficient credit and potential loss of intellectual property rights for those with less power. Junior faculty or students may feel pressured to contribute if they think their participation is linked to promotion and tenure or being able to progress in an academic program. Senior faculty have the responsibility to create a professional relationship that does not disadvantage either party in a student–faculty authorship team. Senior faculty must be able to balance their scholarship interests against the rights of students (Oddi & Oddi, 2000).

Unethical authorship practices, such as excluding those who deserve credit and giving credit when no contribution was made ("gift" authorship), are common. Order of authorship and disagreements about the extent of each contribution are common reasons for disputes and often result in irreparably damaged professional relationships. In some cases, the disputes lead to retractions of publications, and the retraction rate in nursing publications grows each year (Al-Ghareeb et al., 2018).

Ethical publishing practices take commitment from each person on the team and ongoing discussion during the project. A clear understanding at the project start of authorship criteria, the benefits and challenges of coauthorship, and the special challenges when a power differential between authors exists can facilitate ethical publishing practices by encouraging open and collegial discussion among authors.

## Strategies to Address Coauthorship Challenges

Spending time with potential coauthors at the beginning of the project by discussing partnership boundaries may mitigate challenges in coauthorship. Establishing clear expectations, familiarizing the team with differing disciplinary perspectives about any aspect of authorship, acknowledging the power dynamics, and deciding what ongoing effective communication will look like are examples of partnership boundaries (Bergwerk et al., 2022; Conn et al., 2015; Smith & Master, 2017).

After an open and honest discussion about coauthorship with the team, creating formal written agreements goes a long way toward minimizing conflicts later on. Some important considerations include how author credit will be determined, responsibilities and deadlines for the project, and any copyright considerations. The Contributor Roles Taxonomy (more commonly known as CreDIT) is an excellent guide to typical manuscript contributions. Another helpful resource is the authorship grid (Phillippi et al., 2018), which helps define specific contributions from each author and establish the order of authorship. Authorship policies and standardized practices facilitate clear communication about publication, and there is a pressing need for the nursing profession and institutions to develop and implement faculty–student authorship guidelines (Eiswirth & Fry, 2023).

## Knowing Your "Authorial Self"

Being able to successfully write with others means you first need to know who *you* are as an author. Writing is a developmental process. Knowing the type of writing support that will be most beneficial to you is an important part of your growth as a writer. Writing support can be tailored to your needs. One type of support may be very structured, in that a mentor provides detailed guidance about what to do and then shares examples of what good writing looks like. Another type can be a little less structured, in that a mentor reviews and edits your texts, and you learn about writing from the edits. The most interactive type of support occurs when you and a mentor discuss and write collaboratively (González-Ocampo & Castelló, 2018). You may have a chance to use all these strategies throughout your manuscript development. Knowing the types of writing support you need and when you need them is part of your professional development. Do you prefer to look at an example to try and model your writing after it? Or do you prefer to synchronously cowrite in front of the same computer (or legal pad)? Or a combination of both, depending on the type of manuscript?

Academic writing can be formal and highly structured, allowing almost no room for a personal or professional perspective. Or it can be writing that welcomes the author's personal or professional perspective, also known as the author's "voice." Think of your voice as the way you communicate your message (or tell your story) to your intended audience. What type of details or metaphors do you include? Your choice of words, phrases, or metaphors is uniquely yours. Do you tend toward travel metaphors that talk about anticipated destinations but that come with unavoidable delays and cancellations or beautiful gardens that come with weeds? Or some other metaphors entirely? The way you put words together (syntax) and your style (formal, conversational, or something in between) contribute to your voice and will develop and change the more you practice writing. Chinn (2017) asserts that an author's clarity about their personal or professional perspectives creates accountability for the work, which is at the heart of good writing.

Your unique perspective as a DNP practitioner with expertise in a specific patient population will be part of your author's voice and will connect you to your audience of other DNP practitioners. As a member of the DNP community, you have a common frame of reference with your audience. Of course, the audience's level of knowledge will vary, but you are aware of what their baseline knowledge would be and why the topic you are writing about is important to practice for the DNP. Developing your voice as a writer becomes an important part of your academic identity within the academic community, and you can think of it as a work in progress! Staying current with knowledge by attending conferences, reading widely, and interacting with others in the discipline; incorporating the knowledge engagingly into the classes you teach; seeking guidance on submitting conference presentations and journal submissions; and contributing and networking with your professional organizations all will form a firm foundation for your author's voice. That voice does not develop in solitary but instead grows from the collective input from many others.

## Understanding Your Publishing "Why"

Scholarly writing and publishing are intense work, and having a clear idea of why you are doing it, known as your publishing "why," will help you stay motivated. Specifically, why do you wish to publish? It is often helpful to clarify the values guiding your academic work and identify the values that you most identify with. You can find lists of values to choose from in multiple online or print resources. Clark and Sousa's (2018) "Values in Academic Work" is an extremely helpful resource.

Once you've done one of the values clarification exercises, you may find reasons for publishing that resonate with you. Do you feel a sense of responsibility to improve health care or education by making your work visible? Or for you, the value may be a better fit under stewardship for the profession. You may feel a sense of personal fulfillment at practicing to the full extent of your education. Publication of your work is part of the full extent of your education so that others can benefit from your work. The American Association of Colleges of Nursing (2021) advanced-level domain 4 competencies call for advancing the scholarship of nursing, and dissemination as an important part of the competency. Take some time to think about your values, as being clear on them will help motivate you in the writing process.

## Is Your Motivation Internal or External?

Have you ever had to motivate yourself to write your DNP project report, a couple of pages for your nursing program self-study, or even a few book paragraphs like this one on self-motivation? Motivation is the driving force that helps us achieve small and large goals. Strong external driving forces may be events such as deadlines for completing your DNP project. If you miss that deadline, graduation may be denied, so the consequence is harsh. With so much time, energy, and money invested in the DNP program, such a consequence would no doubt result in some guilt and shame over not graduating.

On the other hand, meeting the deadline for DNP project completion brings significant positive consequences. Graduation, recognition from family, friends, and colleagues, and potential career advancement are all strong external motivators. For the graduate, gratification and pride in program completion often create the confidence to know that similar difficult events can be successfully tackled in the future.

Once you have graduated and perhaps started in a faculty role, a strong external driving force for scholarly publishing is often further career advancement. There may be significant consequences (e.g., lack of promotion) for not publishing. To get promoted, you comply with that strong external motivator. In time, you undoubtedly will develop a deeper appreciation for publishing your work when you see that it strengthens your values of improving health care, connecting with colleagues, and adding to the scholarly, nursing-focused literature. That appreciation shifts your motivation from external to internal.

However, self-motivation for writing can take time to develop. During your early professional career, self-motivation may be in the early developmental stages. What can you, as an early career nursing faculty member, do to move toward your internal motivation for writing?

To move toward a time when writing becomes more internally than externally motivated, writing mentors can be a valuable resource. The right type of feedback from a writing mentor can move you toward internal motivation. The feedback should be a sincere attempt to help you meet expectations for your writing and help you be successful. Feedback can help you expand your understanding or initiate an interest in topics you haven't thought about. The right type of feedback has a way of moving you gently toward internal motivation, sometimes without you even noticing that it is happening. As you build positive experiences with your writing, you'll aim for more of them because they are rewarding and self-reinforcing.

Many mentors suggest integrating writing as a daily habit to keep you moving toward your writing goals. Forming a daily writing habit requires nurturing, time, and being gentle with yourself when rocky weeks of work or personal responsibilities need priority. If only the habit could take hold in 21 days! We would all have published articles and books galore. The daily habit will help remodel your brain, moving you toward becoming a writer. Think of the habit as nurturing an infant, progressing to a child, blossoming during adolescence, and then maturing as an adult. While your writing habit won't take 21 years to mature, it will take infinite patience to develop fully, and in the process will bring you both joy and heartache.

A writing mentor can guide you in recognizing your strengths and weaknesses and work with you on a plan for improving those weaknesses. As you do the work necessary to improve, your level of control over your writing strengthens, and with it your pride in yourself and a shift toward internal motivation. Long-term and short-term goals move you toward intrinsic motivation, as your sense of accomplishment grows once they are completed. A short-term goal can be as simple as writing an outline of your manuscript sections. If you build in small rewards for each goal met, the writing process becomes much more pleasurable.

A writing mentor can also help identify other writers who can help you become more productive. We (the authors) have all spent a lot of writing time in isolation and then realized how writing with others led to increased pleasure and productivity. Can counseling provide tools to help with success in writing? Absolutely. Some faculty may benefit from seeking cognitive behavioral therapy from a licensed professional to help squash those negative thoughts and work on mindfulness practices that support writing.

There may be times when the external motivators take an opposite turn. For instance, you may enjoy writing segments for newsletters voluntarily. Your volunteerism is fulfilling because it feels altruistic. But if you start getting paid for the writing, your mind may reframe the writing as work, and with it higher expectations, stress, and a negative association.

With the multiple expectations placed on a new faculty member, writing frequently falls to the bottom of the to-do list. After all, teaching and service obligations are time-sensitive, and you have to show up and get them done. If you're not careful, they will easily fill up all your working hours, and writing is pushed aside. In addition to time constraints, the "publish-or-perish" mentality can lead to negative thoughts about writing, allowing anxiety and the infamous and (ubiquitous!) imposter syndrome monster to creep in. Developing strategies to counteract negative self-talk will serve you well throughout your career, as that inner critic is always hovering in the background, ready to pounce every time you get ready to try a new project.

## Closing Scenario

Dr. Avila recently met one of the senior faculty members during a committee meeting, and they chatted briefly about scholarly writing. They followed up with each other shortly thereafter to explore the possibility of working together as writing partners. Their discussion didn't end in collaboration because it let them know the timing wasn't right for them to work together. Here's how the conversation went:

The senior faculty says to Dr. Avila, "You had mentioned that you were looking for a writing partner, and I'm also looking for a partner. I thought it would be a great idea if we started by discussing our wishes, fears, and concerns regarding publishing and seeing how we can work together. When I think about my wishes for a partnership in publishing, I'm looking for someone who is very knowledgeable of the research process and who may be able to look at issues in my manuscript that demonstrate poor connection or poor logic or just a lack of clarity. Since I'm very busy, I don't want the process to be time-consuming. My fears regarding the partnership are that areas in my manuscript that I think are fine are not fine, and my writing partner does not identify the weaknesses. So, when I send it out for peer review, it will get rejected, and I will have to start from scratch. My concerns are that you are a DNP and because I'm a PhD, we have had very different educational backgrounds and our scholarship may not be a good match. But go ahead and tell me about your wishes, fears, and concerns!"

Dr. Avila looks uncomfortable as she says, "I'm hoping for a partner who will provide guidance and support as I develop a manuscript, and who can help me to grow in this new role of a scholar and writer. I fear that I will appear stupid or dumb to my partner and that I will not be able to produce a manuscript. My concern is that after hearing what you have just said, I would not be able to provide any help for you as I am not at the level yet to provide the kind of feedback you need. Therefore, this would be a less-than-ideal partnership. I look forward to the time we might be able to collaborate, but I think it is too early in my career to be helpful to someone of your stature. I appreciate that you took the time to speak with me, and it was helpful to talk it through."

Dr. Duran kept her promise to facilitate a group of DNPs interested in publishing their projects for a series of seminars. They meet monthly to develop a manuscript from their DNP project. Dr. Duran is experienced in publishing DNP manuscripts and therefore guides participants through the process of developing a scholarly writing partnership and a coauthorship agreement with sample author roles.

## Establishing Effective Partnerships

To promote effective scholarly writing partnerships, scholarly partners should share their wishes regarding the project outcomes, along with their fears or concerns when working with each other. The next step is determining actions that support the relationship and project outcomes. Each partner then decides if they can respect each other's wishes, fears, and concerns in support of the project (Heinrich, 2008).

Complete documents for establishing the partnership, a coauthorship agreement, and a colleague support agreement are in Appendix A. There are separate agreements for coauthors and colleague supporters, as colleague supporters may hold different roles than coauthors. For example, they could serve as a consultant or developmental editor.

What follows is an example of establishing a partnership between Dr. Avila and Dr. Duran that they developed in the DNP publishing seminar.

## Establishing the Partnership

*Sample Sections (full directions and tables available in appendix)*

**TABLE 3.1** Wishes, Fears, and Needs for Sustaining the Relationship

| Coauthor or Collaborator | Wishes for the Scholarly Partnership | Fears or Concerns | Needs for Sustaining the Relationship |
|---|---|---|---|
| Dr. Avila | Help me grow as a scholar and writer. | That I will appear stupid or dumb and not be able to produce a manuscript | Weekly meetings<br><br>Clear directions about the process<br><br>Clear feedback |
| Dr. Duran | Guide Dr. Avila to a successful publishing experience.<br><br>Help Dr. Avila learn the process so she can work with future students. | That I may not be able to provide the necessary level of support needed due to our demanding schedules | Be able to start and finish the meeting on time<br><br>Transparency about what is helpful |

# Coauthor Writing Agreement

Once you have discussed your wishes, fears, and needs and determined a partnership match, it's time to get specific about scholarship goals and what roles each partner would fulfill. The following tables show Dr. Avila's and Dr. Duran's agreement.

They start by setting out their goals, and Dr. Avila's goal is to produce a first draft in the next 6 weeks. They then discuss the roles each of them will have in developing the draft, based on the following author roles table. You'll get more information in the next chapter about publication worksheets, and this table simply shows you a big-picture view of what is ahead!

*Sample Sections (full directions and tables available in appendix)*

**TABLE 3.2** Sample Author Roles for a DNP Project Manuscript

| Role/Tasks | First Author (New DNP) | Second Author (DNP Former Chair or Faculty Experienced With Publishing DNP Manuscripts) |
|---|---|---|
| | Drafts publication worksheet with guidance from a mentor<br>Identifies audience<br>Focuses purpose<br>Develops slant/perspective<br>Targets potential journals | Guides development of publication worksheet |
| Updates and refines literature review to focused purpose and slant | Searches/synthesizes the literature | Cowrites or provides substantial feedback |
| Theory framework | Revises from DNP report if necessary | Cowrites or provides substantial feedback |

| Role/Tasks | First Author (New DNP) | Second Author (DNP Former Chair or Faculty Experienced With Publishing DNP Manuscripts) |
|---|---|---|
| EBP/QI framework | Revises from DNP report if necessary | Cowrites or provides substantial feedback |
| Reporting framework | SQUIRE | Cowrites or provides substantial feedback |

Other areas of the agreement include the timing of meetings, whether the meetings will be in person or virtual, and the type of feedback each coauthor prefers. For example, Dr. Avila likes to receive direct feedback so that she doesn't feel like she needs to "decode" the message. Dr. Duran also appreciates a direct approach related to what Dr. Avila finds helpful. They also discuss how quickly they can expect responses to each other's emails or phone calls. After achieving the scholarly goals, the coauthors agree to a "closure" meeting to discuss what went well during the partnership and what changes could be made in the future to improve the partnership model.

## Application Exercises

Have you been considering coauthoring a manuscript with a colleague? Now is a great time to try this exercise!

Using the appendix to guide you, try the following:

- Establish a partnership with a colleague.
- Develop a coauthorship agreement with a colleague using the sample author roles grid.

What went well? What didn't go well?

## Chapter Wrap-Up

| Knowledge | Skills | Resources |
|---|---|---|
| Authorship and coauthorship definitions<br><br>Benefits and challenges of coauthorship | Implement AACN Essentials, advanced-level domain 4 competencies: "Advance the Scholarship of Nursing" (4.1). | International Committee of Medical Journal Editors (2022) |
| Ethical concerns related to coauthorship | Lead early discussions to promote transparency in coauthorship.<br><br>Use agreements to establish a coauthor role. | Partnership agreement<br><br>Coauthor writing agreement<br><br>Colleague support agreement |
| Understanding the motivation for writing | Express values about academic writing. | Clark & Sousa (2018) |
| Strategies for successful coauthorship | Use available resources to facilitate transparency about all aspects of the coauthor relationship. | CreDIT taxonomy Authorship grid<br><br>Partnership agreement<br><br>Coauthor writing agreement<br><br>Colleague support agreement |

# References

Al-Ghareeb, A., Hillel, S., McKenna, L., Cleary, M., Visentin, D., Jones, M., Bressington, D., & Gray, R. (2018). Retraction of publications in nursing and midwifery research: A systematic review. *International Journal of Nursing Studies, 81*, 8–13. https://doi.org/10.1016/j.ijnurstu.2018.01.013

American Association of Colleges of Nursing. (2021). *The essentials: Core competencies for professional nursing education.* https://www.aacnnursing.org/Portals/42/AcademicNursing/pdf/Essentials-2021.pdf

Bergwerk, M., Lasman, N., Helpman, L., Rosenzweig, B., Cohen, D., Itelman, E., Gross, R., & Segal, G. (2022). Agreement of authorship for student-faculty collaborative research and publications: A literature review and call for action. *The Israel Medical Association Journal, 24*(11), 768–772.

Chinn, P. L. (2017), Finding your voice and writing well: Situating yourself within your text. *Nurse Author & Editor, 27,* 1–9. https://doi.org/10.1111/j.1750-4910.2017.tb00244.x

Clark, A., & Sousa, B. (2018). Values in academic work. In A. Clark & B. Sousa (Eds.), *How to be a happy academic* (pp. 31–43). SAGE.

Conn, V. S., Ward, S., Herrick, L., Topp, R., Alexander, G. L., Anderson, C. M., Smith, C. E., Benefield, L. E., Given, B., Titler, M., Larson, J. L., Fahrenwald, N. L., Cohen, M. Z., & Georgesen, S. (2015). Managing opportunities and challenges of co-authorship. *Western Journal of Nursing Research, 37*(2), 134–163. https://doi.org/10.1177/0193945914532722

Eiswirth, E., & Fry, A. (2022). Faculty-student authorship: Opportunities and challenges. *Journal of Professional Nursing: Official Journal of the American Association of Colleges of Nursing, 42,* 106–110. https://doi.org/10.1016/j.profnurs.2022.06.009

Eiswirth, E. & Fry, A. (2023). Faculty-student authorship practices in nursing: Cross-sectional study. *Journal of Professional Nursing: Official Journal of the American Association of Colleges of Nursing, 49,* 10–15. https://doi.org/10.1016/j.profnurs.2023.08.003

González-Ocampo, G. & Castelló, M. (2018) Writing in doctoral programs: Examining supervisors' perspectives. *Higher Education, 76* (3), 387–401.

Heinrich, K. (2008). Partnerships: How to make writing collaborations pleasurable and productive. *Nurse Author and Editor, 18*(4), 1–4. https://doi.org/10.1111/j.1750-4910.2008.tb00089.x

International Committee of Medical Journal Editors. (2024). *Recommendations for conducting, reporting, editing, and publishing scholarly work in medical journals.* https://www.icmje.org/recommendations/

Nishikawa, J., Codier, E., Mark, D., & Shannon, M. (2015). Student-faculty authorship: Challenges and solutions. *Nurse Author & Editor, 4*(24), 1–9. https://doi.org/10.1111/j.1750-4910.2014.tb00190.x

Oddi, L. F., & Oddi, A. S. (2000). Student-faculty joint authorship: ethical and legal concerns. *Journal of Professional Nursing: Official Journal of the American Association of Colleges of Nursing, 16*(4), 219–227. https://doi.org/10.1053/jpnu.2000.7829

Phillippi, J. C., Likis, F. E., & Tilden, E. L. (2018). Authorship grids: Practical tools to facilitate collaboration and ethical publication. *Research in Nursing & Health, 41*(2), 195–208. https://doi.org/10.1002/nur.21856

Smith, E., & Master, Z. (2017). Best practice to order authors in multi/interdisciplinary health sciences research publications. *Accountability in Research, 24*(4), 243–267. https://doi.org/10.1080/08989621.2017.1287567

# Appendix A: Partnership Documents

The documents included in the appendix include the following:

- Establishing the partnership
- Coauthor writing agreement
- Colleague support agreement

## Establishing the Partnership Sets the Foundation for Agreements

Developing successful scholarly writing partnerships requires a match between individuals. Potential writing partners must explore whether they will be able to work together, support each other, and commit to the scholarly partnership (Heinrich, 2008). The first step is to discuss and fill out the document titled "Establishing the Partnership." Scholarly partners should share their wishes, fears, and concerns regarding the project, and determine the support needed for each one. These actions will support the relationship and lead to a professional agreement.

### Establishing the Partnership

Each partner

- shares their wishes for the partnership outcomes;
- shares their fears or concerns about the partnership; and
- determines if they can respect the other's wishes, fears, and concerns.

Share your wishes for the outcome of the partnership.

| Name of Coauthor or Collaborator | Wishes for the Outcome of the Partnership |
|---|---|
|  |  |
|  |  |

Share your fears or concerns about the scholarly partnership.

| Name of Coauthor or Collaborator | Fears or Concerns About the Scholarly Partnership |
| --- | --- |
|  |  |
|  |  |

Each partner

- shares what they need to sustain a positive, rewarding scholarly relationship;
- determines if they can meet the writing partner's identified needs; and
- includes the identified needs in the written agreement.

| Name of Coauthor or Collaborator | Support Needed |
| --- | --- |
|  |  |
|  |  |

## Draft Agreement

1. Each partner will contribute to creating the agreement.
2. After reviewing the agreement, each partner must determine if they can commit to the partnership.

Once you have established your partnership, it's time to create either a coauthor agreement (if you are writing together) or a colleague support agreement (if you are not writing together but providing feedback on scholarly activities or other supportive actions).

# Coauthor Writing Agreement

Once you have discussed your wishes, fears, and support needs and determined that you have a coauthoring match, it is time to fill out a coauthor writing agreement. The following sample text and tables can help guide the process:

We have agreed to work together and support each other to meet our scholarship goals. We agree to the following guidelines and to assume the best intentions of each other. This agreement ends after the coauthors have achieved the goals outlined in this agreement.

| Names of Coauthors | Goals to Achieve |
| --- | --- |
|  |  |
|  |  |

We enter this agreement voluntarily, and we can leave the agreement voluntarily. We agree that each member in the partnership meets the criteria of authorship as outlined by the International Committee of Medical Journal Editors authorship criteria. We also agree to the order of authorship. The development of the manuscript will be led by the project leader, who will be the first author.

Coauthors are expected to make contributions as specified.

| Names of Coauthor | Author Order | Specified Contributions to the Manuscript |
| --- | --- | --- |
|  |  | Contribution: |
|  |  | Contribution: |

Adding new coauthors should be made by consensus rather than individual decisions.

Resources used in developing the manuscript and draft sections of the manuscript will be shared through ___________ (e.g., One-Drive or other online storage services).

All coauthors can give presentations of this paper after publication, using the material in the paper and/or data set, providing they reference the paper and their coauthors. The coauthor will also notify the team of these presentations beforehand.

## Communication

Participating individuals agree to regularly scheduled meetings and to return responses as specified (e.g., weekly/monthly email updates, phone calls, or face-to-face meetings):

| Communication Method | Schedule |
|---|---|
|  |  |
|  |  |
|  |  |

Coauthors agree to provide equal discussion time for every individual's contribution to this partnership during the regularly scheduled meetings. Coauthors agree they will not commandeer the meetings by taking more than their share of time to discuss their contributions.

All coauthors agree to reply to emails and phone calls concerning manuscript drafts outlined in the agreement within a reasonable time frame (e.g., 48 hours, or whatever your group decides).

Coauthors may voluntarily remove themselves from this agreement at any point if they no longer have time or disagree with some aspect of a project or paper. The order of authorship will be revised and agreed upon by the consensus of remaining members.

Coauthors agree to not share the ideas of another team member outside the group. Coauthors also agree to not share the ideas of others and claim them as their original work.

## Feedback

Coauthors agree to respect each other's method of receiving feedback (e.g. writing, verbal) that is compassionate and constructive.

| Coauthor | Requested Feedback Style |
| --- | --- |
|  |  |
|  |  |

## Supporting the Relationship

Coauthors agree to support each other in meeting recognized needs to help strengthen the scholarly relationship.

| Coauthor | Support Needs |
| --- | --- |
|  |  |
|  |  |

## Closure

After achieving the scholarly goals, the coauthors agree to a "closure" meeting to discuss what went well during the partnership and what changes could be made in the future to improve the partnership model.

## Conflict of Interest

All coauthors will disclose to the team any real or perceived conflicts of interest related to the specified projects and papers outlined in the agreement.

All coauthors will disclose to the team whether they or any close family members or associates will benefit financially from the specified projects and papers outlined in the agreement.

The following coauthors are a part of the agreement.

| Name of Coauthor | Signature of Coauthor | Date |
| --- | --- | --- |
|  |  |  |
|  |  |  |
|  |  |  |

## Colleague Support Agreement

We have already discussed our wishes, fears, and needs and determined we have a collaborative match that will help us meet our scholarship goals when the situation does *not* include coauthorship. Providing feedback to an author on manuscript drafts would be categorized as colleague support.

We agree to the following guidelines as we work together and always assume the best intentions of each other. This agreement ends after the goals outlined in this agreement have been achieved.

| Name of Colleague | Goals to Achieve |
| --- | --- |
|  |  |
|  |  |

We enter this agreement voluntarily, and we can leave the agreement voluntarily.

Collaborators are expected to make contributions as specified.

| Names of Colleague | Specified Contributions |
| --- | --- |
|  | Contribution: |
|  | Contribution: |

Adding new collaborators should be made by consensus rather than individual decisions.

Any individual collaborator requesting support in writing a manuscript intended for publication must consider the possibility that the other collaborator should be considered for coauthors if the criteria of authorship as outlined by the International Committee of Medical Journal Editors Authorship Criteria is met.

## Communication

Participating individuals agree to the regularly scheduled communication as specified (e.g., weekly/monthly email updates, phone calls, or face-to-face meetings):

| Method of Communication | Schedule |
| --- | --- |
|  |  |
|  |  |
|  |  |

Colleagues have agreed to grant every individual's project or manuscript involved in this collaboration equal time during the regularly scheduled meetings. Colleagues agree they will not commandeer the meetings by taking up the regularly scheduled meeting time to discuss issues outside the meeting focus.

All team members agree to reply to emails and phone calls concerning projects and manuscript drafts outlined in the agreement within a reasonable time frame as agreed on by the group.

Team members may voluntarily remove themselves from this agreement at any point if they no longer have time or disagree with some aspect of a project or paper.

Team members are free to develop their collaborations for a different project or manuscript. They agree to not share the ideas of another team member outside the collaborative team and agree to not use the ideas of others and claim them as their original work.

## Feedback

Collaborators agree to respect each other's method of receiving feedback (e.g. writing, verbal) that is compassionate and constructive.

| Names of Collaborators | Style of Feedback |
| --- | --- |
|  |  |

## Supporting the Relationship

Collaborators agree to support each other in meeting needs that would help to strengthen the scholarly relationship.

| Coauthor | Support Needs |
| --- | --- |
|  |  |
|  |  |

## Closure

After achieving goals, colleagues agree to a closure meeting to discuss what went well during the project and what changes could be made in the future.

## Conflict of Interest

All members will disclose any real or perceived conflicts of interest related to specified projects and papers outlined in the agreement.

All members will disclose whether they or any close family members or associates will benefit financially from the specified projects and papers outlined in the agreement.

We agree to the colleague support agreement.

| Name | Signature | Date |
| --- | --- | --- |
|  |  |  |
|  |  |  |
|  |  |  |

# CHAPTER 4

# Unleashing the Publication Potential of Your DNP Project

## Objectives

- Explain essential elements of transforming a DNP report into a manuscript.
- Describe a DNP project that launched a faculty QI project.
- Summarize essential scholarly writing skills.
- Assess your scholarly writing skills.

## Opening Scenario

Dr. Avila says to her mentor, "I've been using my afternoon writing time to draft out the first part of my manuscript. Hanging a "Please Do Not Disturb" sign on my door works well, and I'm able to concentrate. I also started the online writing workshop and received some feedback. I found out that properly citing my sources, critical appraisal, and synthesis are areas I need to improve on, and the workshop facilitators gave us some resources to help with those skills. I'm still a little confused about whether I need to include my former DNP committee chair or other committee members on the manuscript and what things I need to do to turn it into a manuscript. I keep hearing different things from my former classmates about the whole process. I want to do the right thing, but I'm not quite sure what that is." Dr. Duran reassures Dr. Avila that she'll assist her through the process and tells her that she may often hear many misperceptions about publishing in academia. Because of the misperceptions and seemingly unlimited number of "rules," it's important to have someone who is experienced in academic publishing guiding the way.

## Myths and Misperceptions That Keep You Stuck and Unpublished

Undoubtedly, you are extremely proud of your DNP project. The time and energy you invested were significant, and completion means you are ready to graduate. But (unfortunately) it doesn't mean your project report is ready to be published. New DNP graduates frequently believe that publishing their work is a fairly straightforward process after the report is completed, but that's not the case. Taking your work from a project report to a manuscript can be extremely demanding of your time and effort. But don't let that discourage you! For most academic authors, the result of seeing their work published is well worth the effort.

First, let's make sure you can separate the myths and misperceptions from the truth. Here are some common misperceptions that can keep you stuck and unpublished:

- Once the report is finished, it's "almost ready" to be published.

- The report should stay "as is." After all, that's what was approved and blessed by your committee. If you change it, the value would be undermined. You would need their permission to make changes such as editing or rearranging content.

- You did the work of the project, so you should be able to prepare a manuscript for publication without any help.

- You have to add your chair and committee as coauthors because they helped develop the project.

## Transitioning From Report to Manuscript

If you thought anything on the list was a true statement, you have a lot of company. Let's take a closer look at the reality of what needs to be done to turn your report into a manuscript. Determining how to transform your academic paper into a potentially publishable manuscript can be challenging, to say the least. But following a few structured and time-tested steps will help you toward the publication finish line. The following information summarizes recent literature on publishing DNP projects, often from the perspective of nursing journal editors (Carter-Templeton, 2015; Morton & Nerges, 2020; Sebach & Shellenbarger, 2020) and our own editorial and teaching experience. For a helpful table outlining the differences between an academic paper and a manuscript, see Morton and Nerges (2020).

Start by identifying one objective or purpose, from the possibly multiple objectives reported in your academic project. Take some time to think about which purpose will contribute to the body of knowledge that is already available. If it will not contribute anything different, you would need to be able to define why anyone would want to read it. It's important to be able to answer the "so what?" question about your manuscript. Being able to answer the "so what?" question is a process that may take some thinking and discussion and is a very important step to move to publication. "So what" questions are those questions that ask "Why does this matter?" Of course, you can approach that question from many angles. Here are two examples: The work provides a new perspective on an issue or it is a solution to a common problem. If you can define why it would matter to a larger audience, chances are your manuscript will be publishable.

With your project report whittled down to one focus, your literature review will need to be further synthesized and shortened, and the overall reference list will also end up being much shorter than what was included in your report. It is always a good idea to see if the literature review needs updating, especially if 6 months or more have gone by since you wrote your project report. If you have shifted focus slightly on any aspect of the report, you may need to do a more extensive review to make sure you have identified current and relevant literature.

Concurrently with thinking about a more focused topic, it is common to review journals that might be appropriate for your manuscript. Think about the readers of the selected journal and whether your topic would appeal to them. Nurse practitioners who have completed DNP projects may have topics that are not directly transferable to other health care professionals such as registered nurses, physicians, or pharmacists. Selecting a journal requires reviewing the journal's mission, information readership, types of topics covered, and accepted manuscripts. This will inform you of the journal's general audience (readers). Should you find a similar article already published in your selected topic, consider reframing it or building on the already published article. Citing similar articles from the journal lets the editor know you have done the background work when selecting the best journal for your manuscript. In Chapter 5, we'll dive more deeply into how to choose a journal for your manuscript.

DNP project reports typically include more direct quotes than are warranted for a manuscript. When used in a manuscript, direct quotes may provide an impression to journal reviewers that original thinking and synthesis are lacking. Use of direct quotes in scientific health care literature should be limited and reserved for the definition of concepts or measures, seminal research findings, or referencing an item word for word from a survey.

In addition to these changes, the potential audience will shift from your faculty to a larger audience of readers or the chosen journal. Each journal has its own set of guidelines and specific details, such as section headings, referencing style, and table or figure layout, that must be integrated into your manuscript.

In settling on one focus from the few that may have been in your project report, you will probably find you need to rearrange or edit some of the content that no longer addresses your new purpose. Don't let that make you nervous! A common misperception is that you cannot rearrange or remove any content, but that isn't true. Rearranging and removing content is an important step toward

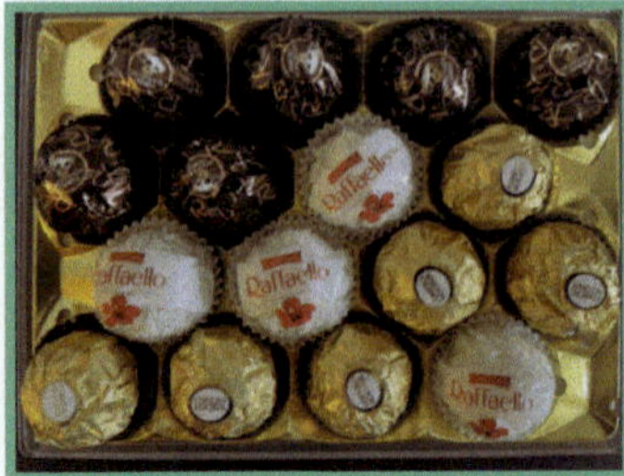

Original box of chocolates

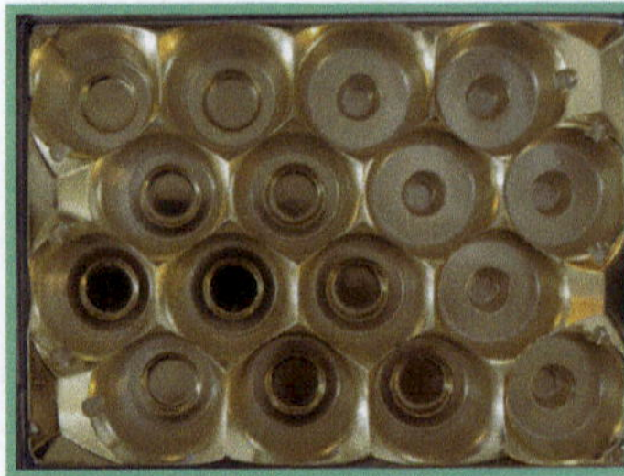

All chocolate removed from the box

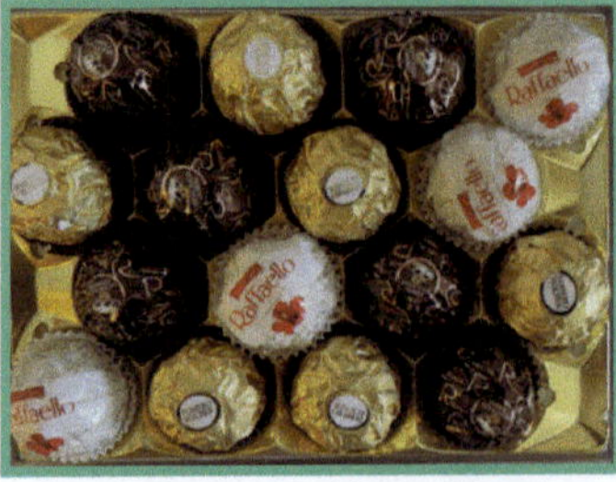

Same chocolates, different arrangement

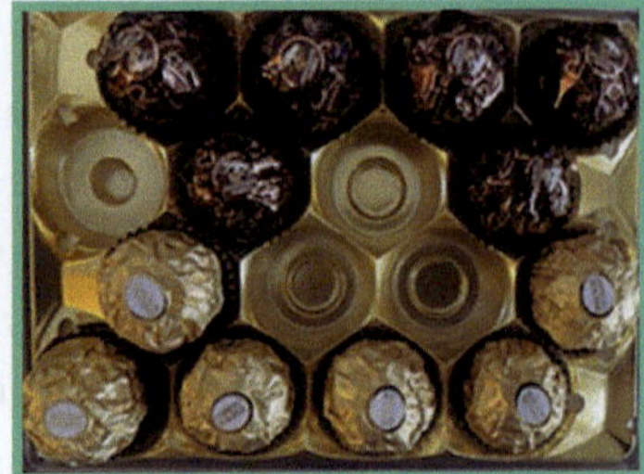

Same chocolates, but fewer of them

**FIGURE 4.1** Rearranging the chocolate exercise in pictures

publication. If it seems like you will be changing the content too dramatically to remain true to your original project, consider the following activity. We call it the "rearranging the chocolate" exercise. Take a picture of a small box of chocolates and the way they are arranged, and then take them out of the box. Once they are out of the box, replace them in any order you choose. You may also choose to leave some of them out. The arrangement has changed, but the essential elements of what is in the box are the same (see Figure 4.1). Think of your rearranged DNP project report in the same way.

## From Rearranging Chocolate to Rearranging Your DNP Report

If you were able to get some extra energy by eating the chocolates after you rearranged them, that's great! Let's use that energy to take a look at your DNP project report and fill in Table 4.1.

**TABLE 4.1** Idea Prompts

| Idea Prompts (Based on SQUIRE Guidelines) | Your DNP Project |
| --- | --- |
| What was the local problem you described? Why was it important to your patient population or to the facility where the project was completed? | |
| What was the purpose of the project? | |
| How does it fit into what is already published on the topic? *What new perspective or problem-solving approach might you suggest?* | |
| What frameworks, models, and/ or theories did you use? | |
| What was the QI process? | |
| What was the outcome? | |

Were you able to identify a new perspective or problem-solving approach? If so, you've begun to identify your "so what" question. Usually, this will take some discussion with colleagues and mentors, as well as updating yourself on what is in the literature. Start thinking and brainstorming, and as we move to the next chapter (where you'll work on a publication worksheet), you'll have some ideas to pursue.

Often, "lessons learned" are an important outcome. While it may seem as if some lessons learned are so obvious, they are not worth mentioning, if they help others think through a project, they *are* worth mentioning. For example, the referral of students being seen at a university student health center to cost-effective health promotion programs on a university campus depends on those programs being available. But sometimes the programs are implemented but then are not sustainable because of funding, and suddenly they are unavailable. A project using best practice guidelines for the treatment of obesity could not implement the guidelines fully because university programs were no longer available (Salcido & Monsivais, 2016). Dependency on other departments or facilities is often underappreciated when implementing guidelines, and considering this before starting a project may save you from some (not all, unfortunately!) frustration.

## A DNP Project That Launched a Faculty QI Project

There are times when your project may serve as a launch pad for another project. Here is a conversation with a faculty member being mentored and her mentor describing that process.

### A Conversation With Dr. Karim Singh (Faculty Being Mentored About Publication)

When I was a fairly new faculty member, I approached Dr. Leslie Robbins to seek her advice about my thoughts that students in my online graduate courses were feeling stressed and a little disconnected from me as their faculty. She expertly guided me to make the connection between my DNP project and the current situation. My DNP project involved creating a video that established a connection between providers and patients (and their families) in the emergency department waiting room at a local hospital. The video provided them with information about what would be happening and introduced them to the people who would be caring for them during their visit. We found that the video helped them wait more patiently and not feel so stressed. And they were more comfortable when called back when it was their turn as they recognized the providers who had been on the video.

Dr. Robbins asked if my online students who were stressed and feeling disconnected might benefit from a video that provided information about the course and helped them get to know the instructor. I immediately saw the potential to decrease stress and anxiety in this different audience and decided to explore the idea. I went back to review my original project write-up to pull out key ideas. Part of my DNP project involved taking an online course to learn best practices in using video media. I increased my skill set quite a bit as I learned about video time length, scripting the narrative, using nature scenes to produce a calming effect, ADA requirements with closed captioning, and a long list of other items necessary to create a professional-looking video.

I decided to investigate ways to use a video to introduce myself to them so that they would feel more connected to me and the course. I did a little background investigation and a brief literature review. I identified a framework called the community of inquiry that has been shown to increase student engagement and connectedness in online courses. One key area of the framework is teacher presence, which engages students and decreases their stress. Teacher presence would be increased if students could get to know the faculty member through an online introductory video. I realized I could tap into the skills I had gained in video production to create an introductory online video to connect with my students.

I made an appointment with our video experts on campus to find out what I needed to do next. They were very helpful and listened when I shared my vision for my introductory video. I wanted to make sure it adhered to best practices, and I wanted it to be true to who I am as a clinician and educator. Portraying my authenticity was important to me, as I wanted students to know I was approachable and had their best interests at heart. I scripted a narrative, and in remembering the calming effects of nature, used the beautiful campus as background scenes for some of the videos. I also used some scenes of me working in the clinic so that students could get to know me as a clinician as well as an educator.

Once I had used the video in an online course for a semester, I collected student feedback, and it was overwhelmingly positive. They expressed that they appreciated seeing me on the video so that I was more than a voice or a name on the discussion board. They said they felt more connected because they knew my background, and this made them less anxious about their future interactions with me.

Because connecting with online students is such an important skill, Dr. Robbins suggested I present this project at a national meeting. With her guidance, I developed a presentation about the project and then presented it at a national meeting. The experience was so affirming, and there were many questions about the process and so much interest in doing the same thing. Many programs were transitioning to an online format and striving to improve the online environment. We had so much positive feedback that I came home energized and wanted to take the next step of publishing it.

She guided me in reviewing the original concepts in my DNP project to use those as the backbone of the publication. Essentially, we'd be deconstructing what was done originally and reconstructing it for a new audience. But through the reconstruction for a new audience, best practices of video production would be maintained, as would the goals of increasing connectedness and decreasing stress for the audience.

I worked to transition my presentation worksheet to a publication worksheet. In deconstructing the main concepts in my original project, I was able to look at how similar ideas were being transitioned to a different audience. With feedback from Dr. Robbins, I developed the publication worksheet. As I drafted it, I wasn't sure I was being entirely objective as I had been working so closely with the material. She suggested sending drafts out to faculty who were experienced in publishing and asking for feedback. I was nervous about receiving feedback from colleagues as I wasn't sure how I would receive negative comments because it's hard not to take them personally. But I know that's the best way to get a strong manuscript, so I was willing to do it. Fortunately, they provided kind and constructive feedback, and I felt my manuscript was improved by their suggestions. I double-/triple-checked my citations and made sure all my references were current. As I reread the manuscript (many times!), I realized how much of my DNP project was beneficial in my faculty role. It is interesting that even though the publication has a different audience than my DNP project, I could transition the important skills I learned to my new audience to achieve similar outcomes of increasing connectedness and decreasing stress by using a video. I realized it was also beneficial across all levels of faculty who teach online, and creating the manuscript was a way to disseminate this important information. With a combination of high hopes and more than a little anxiety, I finally submitted my manuscript.

Honestly, I felt deflated when I got the comments back after the first submission. Because I didn't know how to interpret them, I consulted Dr. Robbins. She reassured me they were things that could be easily addressed, and they did not mean the manuscript was rejected or that I wasn't a good writer. I learned how to create a reviewer response table to address the comments. After the second submission, the manuscript came back with a few more suggestions for revisions. This time, I understood that requests for revisions are generally a good thing because they mean the editor is trying to move the manuscript toward publication. And, because I had already created one response table, it was much easier the second time around to revise. The manuscript was then accepted and published (Singh & Robbins, 2020). While I was surprised at the time and attention needed to write a manuscript, the effort and hard work faded into the background as the goal of publishing was fulfilled!

## A Conversation With Dr. Leslie Robbins (Publication Mentor)

Dr. Singh's project provides an example of using a skill developed during her DNP project and applying it to a quality improvement project when she became a faculty member. During her DNP project, she created a video to play in the waiting room of a local hospital. The project arose from the ubiquitous problem of long waiting times, and patients who were stressed and angry by the time they were seen. The video provided information and introduced those waiting to people who would be taking care of them during their visit. For the patients and their families, having the video playing decreased their stress and made them more comfortable and in a better frame of mind to listen because they recognized the providers from the video and understood everyone was doing everything possible for their care.

The project was a resounding success, and patients evaluated the video very positively in terms of decreasing their stress and making them feel welcomed. One of the important things Dr. Singh did was use actual representatives from the community on the video. In this case, she used her own family and friends rather than professional actors. This created an immediate connection with her waiting room audience and made them feel welcomed as the audience shown was an authentic representation of the community.

Shortly after she began teaching, Dr. Singh approached me about ways to decrease stress and increase the engagement of students in her online classes. She knew learning outcomes were often dependent on how connected the students felt to the course and their faculty members. We brainstormed, researched, and discussed ideas. Just as the hospital waiting room video decreased stress and made the patients and families feel welcomed, we realized an introductory video from the course faculty was an excellent means of providing those benefits to students in an online class. Dr. Singh supported the new project idea with evidence from the literature showing teacher presence in an online course increases engagement and improves learning outcomes, and she pursued creating an introductory online video.

It seemed the skills she gained in video production had just been waiting to be transferred to a new project! The key concepts in production remained the same even though the audience was now very different. She was moving from an audience of patients and families waiting in a hospital waiting room to students in an online class. But the core elements of producing the video would be the same. Those core elements would be video timing, using scenes from nature, and depicting her authenticity as an educator and clinician. Her background as a clinician is a very important part of what she brings to the educator role, and the video showed a clip of her in the clinic seeing patients. This allowed students to connect with both their instructor and their future, as they could visualize themselves in their future clinician role.

A large part of what I did during the process was make connections to ideas and resources. Once we connected that the skills for video production could be transferred to a new audience, I suggested she contact campus experts with the equipment for video production to help her begin creating the video. After the video was used in the class, I helped her make connections between the feedback from students and feedback from the hospital waiting room about the video. My longer experience in academia and publishing also allowed me to identify an appropriate conference to present her project, facilitate writing the manuscript after the presentation, and highlight how the essence of her DNP project was maintained and achieved the goals of increasing connections and decreasing stress even though the audience was different. I hope that this discussion of how Dr. Singh evolved her DNP project into a faculty QI project and then developed a manuscript provides useful tips for those mentors and mentees who wish to do the same thing.

# Defining Essential Scholarly Writing Skills

If you find that properly citing sources, critical appraisal, and synthesis are areas for improvement, you have a lot of company. The publication potential of your manuscript will often depend heavily on your scholarly writing skills, and new DNP graduates frequently need support and mentorship to guide the publication process (Ayala et al., 2022; DeCoux Hampton & Chafetz, 2020).

## Scholarly Writing Skills

The concept of "scholarly writing skills" is a broad one, and it's a good idea to make sure we're using the same definition. Essential writing skills for professional journal manuscripts include correct citation, critical appraisal, and succinct presentation (synthesis) of content, so we'll use those concepts to define scholarly writing skills. Are you interested in assessing your skills? You can self-assess with the CUNY Assessment Test in Writing (CATW) Student Handbook (City University of New York, 2012). The handbook is extremely helpful and will allow you to get an idea of areas for improvement.

If you were fortunate enough to have developed your writing skills while in your DNP program, you may have done very well on the assessment. Some programs have strategies for intentionally helping students develop writing skills through the curriculum. The strategies may have involved other departments such as the library or writing center in collaboration with program faculty, sequencing assignments throughout the program, or providing support from an expert who has experience with nursing scholarship (Kilmer et al., 2023; Woodward & Hirsch, 2023). However, more commonly you may not have had a chance to develop your writing skills, leaving new graduates to wonder about the writing skills that will help move the project report to publication. With that in mind, we'll provide an overview and resources related to the main skills of scholarly writing: citations, critical appraisal, and synthesis.

## Citations

You may find the online resource "Good Citation Behavior" (Web of Science Academy-Clarivate™, 2021) useful in helping develop your citation skills. If properly quoting is a challenge, look at "Using Quotations in Scientific Writing" (University of Washington, 2014).

## Critical Appraisal

Critical appraisal involves assessing the validity of research, which allows for making practice decisions on the best evidence available to provide the best outcomes possible. Validity assessment involves evaluating the research design, methods, analysis, and findings.

The quality of the evidence is frequently not considered when making practice recommendations (Yao et al., 2021). Good quality evidence derived from research that is carefully constructed and conducted leads to a higher degree of certainty that the desired outcome will occur. On the other hand, weaker evidence provides a much lower degree of certainty that the desired results will be achieved. You'll find appraisal tools readily available from the Center for Evidence-Based Practice (Johns Hopkins Medicine) (n.d.), Centre for Evidence-Based Medicine (University of Oxford) (n.d.), and JBI (n.d).

## Synthesis Writing

Synthesis is a difficult writing skill, and it takes ongoing practice. Key features of synthesis include reporting information from varied sources using different phrases than in the original studies, organizing the information so areas where the information overlaps are easily apparent, and interpreting the sources so the reader can understand them in depth (Jamieson, 1999).

While learning the basics of synthesis and then practicing it can take time and effort, this skill can provide extraordinary benefits. Information synthesis is a means for identifying new ideas, which often provides a foundation for new perspectives about a topic. New perspectives about the topic often lead to the creation of a new model or framework (Torraco, 2005) that builds the evidence foundation in the nursing profession. There are multiple sources for professional development with synthesis writing. One of the most comprehensive resources identified is Darowski et al. (2022), who combine in-class discussion with an online tutorial. The online tutorial consists of seven short, engaging videos (Darowski et al., 2016). When an in person group activity is needed, one effective teaching-learning strategy is "Don't Be a Serial Citer. Synthesize!" (Monsivais & Robbins, 2020). Drew University On-Line Resources for Writers (n.d.) provides an excellent overview and clear examples.

Have you been hesitant to combine original ideas from others and use them to build a framework for something different? Or simply to suggest something new? We offer permission to do that with an "Author Prescription to Create Something Different!"

## Author Prescription

Your name ________________

Synthesize and create something different when you write. Remember that your evaluation of the literature, identification of a knowledge gap in which to situate your work, and use of a particular theory are all ways that count as original thought in academic writing.

Once your paper is complete, an excellent resource to help you evaluate your work is the Scientific Writing Assessment by DeCoux Hampton (2020). The scoring rubric is accompanied by detailed explanatory criteria that enable the user to objectively assess multiple components of a scientific paper. Examples of what is included in the assessment are fundamental skills related to writing mechanics such as grammar, punctuation, and formatting; information literacy and integrity such as the use of primary sources and paraphrasing; and conceptualization and critical analysis that contribute meaningfully to the literature.

You can use the rubric to assess your own work, or you can ask a trusted colleague to review your work against the rubric for you. If you choose to combine both your own and a colleague's assessment, any discussion of differing viewpoints would provide an excellent learning opportunity for both you and your colleague. While punctuation and formatting standards tend to be concrete, judgments about critical appraisal of primary sources and synthesis of evidence tend to be more abstract and therefore lend themselves to more discussion.

Take another look at the myths and misperceptions and decide how you would answer them after reading this chapter:

- Once the report is finished, it's "almost ready" to be published.
- The report should stay "as is." After all, that's what was approved and blessed by your committee. If you change it, the value will be undermined. You would need their permission to make changes such as editing or rearranging content.
- You did the work of the project, so you should be able to prepare a manuscript for publication without any help.
- You have to add your chair and committee as coauthors because they helped develop the project.

## Closing Scenario

Dr. Avila meets with Dr. Duran to update her and says, "The feedback I've been getting from my workshop shows that I'm improving my scholarly writing. I'm doing much better with citations and critical appraisal since I started paying attention and using the tools available. I'm still struggling with synthesis, but I've been doing the online video tutorials and getting a better idea of what I need to do. I spoke with my former chair about whether I'm supposed to put her or my committee on any manuscripts, and she told me there is not a rule that says I need to do that. But she would be willing to coauthor as second author if I wanted her to. We set up a time to review my project and brainstorm appropriate perspectives for a manuscript as well as review authorship criteria and use of the authorship grid for specific tasks assigned to each author. I'm very excited to have unlocked the publication potential of my DNP report so that I can transform it into a manuscript!"

# References


Ayala, F. J., DeBoard, E., Waldrop, J., Pereira, K., Oermann, M. H., & Silva, S. G. (2022). Dissemination of Doctor of Nursing practice project findings: Benefits and challenges associated with publishing in healthcare journals. *Nursing Outlook, 70*(6), 846–855. https://doi.org/10.1016/j.outlook.2022.07.011

Carter-Templeton, H. (2015), Converting a DNP scholarly project into a manuscript. *Nurse Author & Editor, 25,* 1–7. https://doi.org/10.1111/j.1750-4910.2015.tb00195.x

Center for Evidence-Based Practice. (n.d.). *Johns Hopkins evidence-based practice model.* Johns Hopkins Medicine. https://www.hopkinsmedicine.org/evidence-based-practice/model-tools

Centre for Evidence-Based Medicine. (n.d.). *Critical appraisal tools.* University of Oxford. https://www.cebm.ox.ac.uk/resources/ebm-tools/critical-appraisal-tools

City University of New York. (2012). *CUNY assessment test in writing (CATW). Student Handbook.* https://www.cuny.edu/wp-content/uploads/sites/4/page-assets/academics/testing/cuny-assessment-tests/test preparation-resources/StudentHandbookCATWWebnew.pdf

Darowski, E. S., Helder, E., & Patson, N. D. (2022). Explicit writing instruction in synthesis: Combining in-class discussion and an online tutorial. *Teaching of Psychology, 49*(1), 57–63. https://doi-org.utep.idm. oclc.org/10.1177/0098628320979899

Darowski, E. S., Patson, N. D., & Helder, E. (2016). *Using synthesis in your writing.* [Video]. YouTube. https://www.youtube.com/playlist?list=PLHIcqvtKwJAzkID-TvEtPqJ2_bSGbsROk

DeCoux Hampton, M. (2020). Scientific writing assessment guide for faculty use. http://links.lww.com/NE/A801. Licensed under a Creative Commons Attribution-NonCommercial-NoDerivatives 4.0 International License.

Drew University On-Line Resources for Writers. (n.d.). *Synthesis writing.* https://users.drew.edu/sjamieso/synthesis.html#literature

Jamieson, S. (1999). Drew University on-line resources for writers. Synthesis writing. https://users.drew.edu/sjamieso/synthesis.htm

JBI (n.d.). *Critical appraisal tools.* https://jbi.global/critical-appraisal-tools

Kilmer, M., Bradley, C., Raines, A., & Blair, D. (2023). Integrating writing throughout the curriculum in Doctor of Nursing practice programs: A collaborative model for success. *The Journal of Nursing Education, 62*(4), 241–248. https://doi.org/10.3928/01484834-20230208-06

Monsivais, D. B., & Robbins, L. K. (2020). Don't be a serial citer. Synthesize! *Nursing Education Perspectives, 41*(1), 65–66. https://doi.org/10.1097/01. NEP.0000000000000419

Morton, P. G., & Nerges, J. (2020). Strategies to turn a graduate school paper into a publishable journal manuscript. *AACN Advanced Critical Care, 31*(4), 371–379. https://doi.org/10.4037/aacnacc2020716

Salcido, M. E., & Monsivais, D. (2016). Screening and management of overweight and obesity in a university student health center. *The Nurse Practitioner,* 41(7), 50–54.

Sebach, A. M., & Shellenbarger, T. (2020). Modifications needed: Additional strategies to transform DNP projects into publishable manuscripts. *Nurse Author & Editor, 30,* 1–8. https://doi.org/10.1111/j.1750-4910.2020. tb00057.x

Singh, K. C., & Robbins, L. K. (2020). Remind me you are real: Creating a self-introductory video for online courses. *Teaching and Learning in Nursing, 15*(3), 195–197.

Torraco, R. J. (2005). Writing integrative literature reviews: Guidelines and examples. *Human Resource Development Review,* 4(3), 356–367. https:// doi.org/10.1177/1534484305278283

University of Washington. (2014). *Using quotations in scientific writing.* Psychology Writing Center. https://psych.uw.edu/storage/writing_center/ quotes.pdf

Web of Science Academy-Clarivate™. (2021). *Good citation behavior.* https://
webofscienceacademy.clarivate.com/learn

Woodward, K. F., & Hirsch, A. (2023). Discipline-specific writing support
in graduate nursing. *The Journal of Nursing Education, 62*(4), 253–256.
https://doi.org/10.3928/01484834-20230104-01

Yao, L., Guyatt, G. H., & Djulbegovic, B. (2021). Can we trust strong recommendations based on low quality evidence? *BMJ (Clinical Research
Edition), 375*, n2833. https://doi.org/10.1136/bmj.n2833

# Appendix B: Writing Resources

Explore the helpful resources that follow:

- Duke Trinity College of Arts and Sciences. Thompson Writing Program: https://twp.duke.edu/twp-writing-studio/
resources-students

- John Wiley & Sons, Inc. (2016). Writing for Publication.
An Easy-to-Follow Guide for Nurses: https://onlineli-
brary.wiley.com/pb-assets/assets/14667657/Writing_for_
Publication-1509467251000.pdf

- Taylor & Francis Group. How to Write and Structure a
Journal Article: https://authorservices.taylorandfran-
cis.com/publishing-your-research/writing-your-paper/
writing-a-journal-article/

- The Ohio State University. College of Arts and Sciences.
Center for the Study and Teaching of Writing. Tips and
Tools: https://cstw.osu.edu/tips-and-tools

- The Writing Center. University of North Carolina at
Chapel Hill. Tips & Tools: https://writingcenter.unc.edu/
tips-and-tools/

- University of Missouri-Kansas City. Graduate Writing
Resources. Apps & Tools for Graduate Students: https://
libguides.library.umkc.edu/gradwriting/apps-tools

# CHAPTER 5

# Finding a Journal for Your Manuscript-in-Progress

## Objectives

- Highlight the benefits of using a publication worksheet to create a focused manuscript.
- Develop a manuscript publication worksheet based on your DNP project.
- Describe the importance of disseminating scholarship in reputable journals.
- Appraise journals for quality criteria.
- Identify possible target journals for your manuscript.

### Opening Scenario

With excitement, Dr. Avila tells her mentor that she's been invited to submit a manuscript for publication in a nursing journal. "The email said the editor had read my previous work and had been very impressed by the topic and that it would be a good match for the journal. They also said there was a discount on the article publication charge if I submitted it in the next 10 days. Do you think I should do this?" Dr. Duran says, "I'm glad you recognize the importance of publishing your work. There are many things to consider when deciding where to submit a manuscript. One of the most important is whether the journal is reputable. I'll share the criteria with you to help you decide whether the journal that sent the invite is reputable, as well as other things to consider when finding a journal match for your manuscript. First, though, let's make sure you have a plan in place for a publication, and we'll start with a publication worksheet."

## Your Manuscript Plan Starts With a Publication Worksheet

A publication worksheet will help you develop a focused idea and plan for your manuscript. Worksheets may seem too basic and synonymous with grammar school, but they work! When we suggest creating worksheets, the reaction from aspiring authors is usually to spend a lot of time trying to figure out how to get out of doing one. Eventually, they'll find it's easier (and less time-consuming) just to create a worksheet from the start.

Even though it seems like your manuscript will be written directly from your DNP project report, much needs to be edited and revised. Without the worksheet, it is too easy to veer off track and lose focus. It's happened to all of us and to every student we have guided to publication. The overwhelming consensus is that the time invested in planning will pay off in a big way. The essential worksheet components we'll discuss are drawn from Heinrich's (2008) *A Nurse's Guide to Presenting and Publishing: Dare to Share.*

---

### Publication Worksheet

*Idea or main topic for the manuscript:*

*Purpose of the manuscript:*

> *What is the new perspective you will bring to the literature about this topic?*
>
>
> *One-sentence description (addresses the topic, purpose, audience, and perspective):*
>
>
> *Possible title ideas:*
>
>
> *Three potential journals listed in order of preference:*

## Drafting Your Publication Worksheet

It seems like there are a lot of blank areas to fill in, but you already have some of the information. First, write down the manuscript idea or main topic. Generally, of course, the idea comes from your DNP project. Here's an example: If your project was about improving adherence to self-management strategies for patients with diabetes and you used Leininger's culture care diversity and universality theory (McFarland & Wehbe-Alamah, 2015) to guide the project, your manuscript idea or main topic might look something like this:

> What family nurse practitioners need to know about cul-
> turally appropriate diabetes self-management strategies

Your manuscript purpose might look something like this:

> Describe a diabetes self-management program guided by
> Leininger's culture care diversity and universality theory.

Take an honest look at how your purpose fits into what is already published on the topic. What new perspective or problem-solving approach might you suggest? In this example, it might be how theory guided the project. It might also be lessons learned with a particular population or a combination of both.

Once you have your perspective, you are ready to create a one-sentence description of the manuscript. Your one sentence should address the topic, purpose, audience, and perspective or slant (Heinrich, 2008). Crafting this sentence takes some practice and may take discussion with colleagues. But once it's in place, the manuscript becomes much easier to write because you have clearly identified what you will be writing about.

Your one-sentence description might look something like this:

> This manuscript will inform readers about implementing standardized guidelines for diabetes self-management and the value of using Leininger's culture care diversity and universality theory to guide self-management strategies.

With a general plan in mind for the manuscript, it's time to brainstorm a title.

## Choosing a Title That Invites Readers Into the Scholarly Conversation

Choosing a title is a very important step in creating your manuscript. You've probably not spent too much time thinking about the impact a title can have. After all, because *you're* interested in the topic, it seems like any title should work because you find the content interesting. But if someone is not familiar with your work, you'll need to convince them it's worth reading. Consider the title as advertising for the content of your work and your chance to attract the reader to read it.

Think about how you decide which articles to read from a PubMed search for papers that you've written for your classes. You're looking for content that matches what you need as background for your paper, and if the title doesn't inform you about the right content, you skim past it without even looking at the abstract. If the title tells you about the content and also sounds interesting to read, what a bonus! Then there's the occasional time that the title is not in the content area you need right then but sounds so interesting you want to read it anyway and you take a slight detour down a reading side road. Now *that's* a good title. (Never be afraid of taking one of those side roads, as they often produce "aha" moments!)

Think of an inviting title as your conversational opener. When you initiate an in-person conversation, you often try to ask an interesting question or comment about something to get the conversation started. Your title can do the same thing if you think of it as a way to bring others scholars into your (scholarly) conversation. You hope they will read and cite your work, increasing the depth of the conversation.

There are some general guidelines for writing titles, and knowing what they are is important. The publication manual of the American Psychological Association (2020) advises being focused and succinct, including important concepts and keywords (e.g., a particular population), and creating a title that engages readers, but they do not set a word limit. While no source prescribes a set number of words, 10–14 words seem to be a common recommendation. But journals have their own guidelines and often allow more words than that. Creating a great title is tougher than it seems at first glance. And the shorter titles are the toughest because they take more work to get them right. However, the work is worth your time because there is evidence shorter titles have a higher number of downloads and citations (Jamali & Nikzad, 2011; Rossi & Brand, 2020). And of course, the title should accurately reflect the content and not deceive readers by promising content that is not there (Monsivais, 2021).

A title that engages readers, while also being informative and fulfilling the word limit, is no easy task. It's also dependent on the discipline, and what might be considered an engaging title in some disciplines may lead those in other disciplines to decide the work is not important because it is perceived as unscholarly (Sword, 2012). Therefore, knowing the readership of the journal is key to crafting your title.

Along with thinking about the content of your title, you also want to consider your "slant" or perspective. A manuscript slant interprets or presents content in line with a special interest (Merriam-Webster, n.d.). It's the point of view or perspective that will engage your reader. What kind of distinct perspective does your manuscript have? Is it a knowledge gap or practical implication? Is there a controversy related to the topic? Was it lessons learned? Are you describing the application of a theory to your project?

Whatever your perspective is, make sure your title showcases your slant. A great title will probably not pop out right as you start drafting your publication worksheet. It's usually an evolving process, so be patient and keep the ideas flowing until the title resonates for you and any other authors working on the manuscript. You'll start with a working title, which might include all elements of the project (your population, type of project, methods, etc.), so it will be very long. Check whether the title includes key terms used in Medical Subject Headings so that it will be easier for others to find in database searches (Langford & Pearce, 2019; Pearce et al., 2018). Keep a running list of ideas as they occur to you and others on your team (or even outside your team) while working on the manuscript.

Titles are broadly categorized into descriptive, declarative, interrogative, or compound. Let's look at examples of each:

- *Descriptive titles*: These are straightforward, describe the content, and are very common in academia. Here's an example:

  Assessing Vaccine Hesitancy Among Pediatric Healthcare Providers (Pope et al., 2022)

- *Declarative or informative titles*: These inform about the outcome of the project, like this example:

  Increasing Human Papillomavirus Immunization in the Primary Care Setting (Taylor et al., 2021)

- *Interrogative titles*: These are question-style titles that ask the reader to consider a point. These are much less frequently used than the first two. This one combines a question with a descriptive title:

  Can Quality Improvement Improve the Quality of Care? A Systematic Review of Reported Effects and Methodological Rigor in Plan-Do-Study-Act Projects (Knudsen et al., 2019)

- *Compound titles*: These are composed of two sections separated by a colon. Historically, nursing seems to have an affinity for compound titles (Diers & Downs, 1994) and does not show signs of stopping. Here are a couple of recent ones:

Practicing Upstream: Race-Based Trauma Care Training for Veteran's Health Administration Nurse Practitioners (Loyd & Scaglione, 2022)

From Bedside to Webside: Telehealth Education for Doctoral Nursing Students (Herrera & Foronda, 2022)

## So Many Journals to Choose From!

With so many journals available, and with a range of considerations when deciding where to submit, the task of targeting a journal can seem overwhelming. Certainly, your topic often narrows down the choices. If you have a nursing education-focused topic or a clinical topic, the journal choices are usually distinct. But after that, things can get confusing. Conlogue et al. (2022) found that participants in their study determined where to submit a manuscript based on the following factors: (a) if the topic fits the scope of the journal; (b) the journals they read; (c) colleague recommendations; (d) if it is listed on PubMed.gov; (e) if it listed on Medline or Web of Science; (f) if it is listed on Journal Citation Reports (JCR), SCImago Journal Rank (SJR), or Journal Author Name Estimator (JANE); (g) if it is listed on Google Scholar; and (h) librarian recommendations.

Those are all great places to start, but there's work to be done after you've identified some possibilities. The first thing to do is investigate the journal's quality criteria. The quality of a journal matters to your scholarly reputation (and to that of your employer). Your publications may have a direct impact on promotion and tenure considerations and may impact grant applications. Grant reviewers may rely heavily on your publications listed to show your knowledge and credibility with the topic. That means you'll want to steer clear of all journals that fall into the "predatory" category.

Check the journal website for information about the journal's policy on query letters. Some journal editors prefer to have the author simply submit the manuscript rather than send a query letter. Because journal guidelines usually are definitive about the journal's scope, and electronic manuscript submission systems allow quick response to authors, it is usually more efficient to simply submit the manuscript.

## Definitions

The Committee on Publication Ethics (COPE, 2019) defines predatory publishing as a

> systematic for-profit publication of purportedly scholarly content (in journals and articles, monographs, books, or conference proceedings) in a deceptive or fraudulent way and without any regard for quality assurance. (p. 3)

Clearly, predatory journals are not where you want to publish your work! Doing some background investigation may be necessary to make sure you find a journal worthy of your manuscript. You can start by assessing a journal's quality indicators using the "Principles of Transparency and Best Practice in Scholarly Publishing." These principles are a collaborative effort of COPE, the Directory of Open Access Journals, the Open Access Scholarly Publishers Association, and the World Association of Medical Editors (2022). Let's look at some of the principles and what they mean as you acquaint yourself with potential journals.

One of the first things to check is the name of the journal, which should be distinctive and not one that is easily confused with another journal. Predatory journals often have names that are very similar to well-known journals, and the idea is to deceive you into thinking it is *the* well-known journal. Make sure to check out the journal name from somewhere you know is reputable (e.g., the Nursing Journal Directory (n.d.), which is a joint service of Nurse Author & Editor and the International Academy of Nursing Editors (INANE)). If it's not there, it may be a good indicator that it's not a nursing journal that you want to be associated with. One of the most visible areas of assessment is the journal's website. It should be well-designed (professional looking) and easy to navigate, and links should be functional. Assessing a journal's website may take some practice, as you may need to review a fair number of reputable journal websites before being able to recognize a predatory journal website. Let's call it "website situational awareness." As an experienced educator or clinician, your radar goes up if something is not right with a student or patient situation. Your experience gives you a basis to make judgment calls about what is normal. Until you have that experience, you are relying on your book knowledge and someone with more experience to get you through. The process of determining whether a journal website and the journal itself is reputable works the same way. We'll give you that book knowledge, but until you are comfortable making the assessment, you should ask an experienced colleague when something is confusing.

As you review a journal website, it should be easy to find the aims and scope, who the target readers are, and the types of manuscripts that can be submitted. Additionally, the publishing schedule and policies for archiving, copyright terms, and licensing information should be visible. Policies related to publication ethics should also be easily available. Examples of ethics policies are those related to authorship, handling complaints and appeals, conflicts of interest, how to access the journal articles (e.g., subscription or pay per view), and article publication fees (COPE et al., 2022).

What about the peer review process? The peer review process remains foundational to the integrity and validity of scientific publications, and a rigorous process is important to maintain this integrity and validity. Promises of quick peer review and quick acceptance should alert you to possible predatory practices. Traditional publishing practices generally set deadlines for peer reviewers to return a review within a certain period (often between 3 to 4 weeks), and the process depends on whether the reviewers can accept the assignment and then meet their deadlines. Peer reviewing is a volunteer activity, often carried out as a professional service because reviewers recognize that their work was published because others took the time to review and provide feedback for them. Busy academics and clinicians do their best to meet their agreed-on deadline for a review but cannot always do so due to the demands of other commitments. Therefore, guarantees of a speedy review should be a red flag of possible predatory practice since it indicates a rigorous review is probably not taking place.

Ownership and management of journals have not traditionally been the concern of new authors but are important matters to review and should be clearly stated on the journal's website. Either a corporate publisher or a professional organization may publish journals. Reputable corporate publishers for nursing and medical journals, for example, include (but not exclusively) Elsevier, Springer, Wiley, and Wolters Kluwer. No doubt, they are immediately familiar to many readers. Society journals are those that you receive as part of your membership in a specialty organization, such as the American Association of Neuroscience Nursing, Society of Trauma Nurses, Association of Rehabilitation Nurses, or nonspecialty organizations such as the National League for Nursing or Sigma. In some cases, you may find a well-known publisher publishes a society journal. If you don't recognize the name of the society or the publisher, you should be able to find information about them on other online resources and verify legitimacy that way. If not, it is most likely an indication that you should not submit your work to the journal.

The editor and editorial boards should be listed with their full names and institutional affiliations, and they should be published scholars in the discipline. You may have to do some investigative work to determine what they have published by searching PubMed or other databases. If the editor or an editorial board member is not a member of the nursing discipline, there should be a clear explanation of their qualifications for the position on the editorial board of a nursing journal.

The journal should be indexed in reputable databases that have quality-control criteria. It can be easy to confuse reputable databases with those that are simply searchable databases. Searchable database examples are Open J-Gate, JournalSeek, and Cross-Ref, and they do not have any quality-control criteria for journals to be included in them. Predatory journals often display these searchable databases proudly on their website, hoping you will think the journals have met some type of standard to be included and that the inclusion is meaningful. On the other hand, reputable databases such as ERIC, Web of Science, SCOPUS, EBSCO, MEDLINE, PubMed, and CINAHL do have an application process. The journal must demonstrate adherence to publication best practices to earn a listing as part of the reputable database. Since criteria for inclusion include a minimum publication time and a certain number of peer-reviewed articles, it is possible that a new journal that is just getting started is reputable but does not yet meet those indicators.

## How Much Emphasis Should You Put on Journal Metrics?

Citation-based metrics are numerous and can be very confusing. Choosing a journal solely based on the journal's calculated citation impact scores provides mixed messaging to junior authors. Sometimes understanding these types of metrics can make you feel like you are in a horror movie and are running down the hallway and the door you are trying to reach keeps getting farther and farther away. What a cruel world! We don't recommend spending valuable time understanding these types of calculations if they create a stress response. University librarians have a wealth of knowledge in this area and are an invaluable resource if you need help understanding journal metrics. Here's some interesting background about the whole situation.

During the first quarter of the 1900s, university librarians were tasked to collect journals most relevant to specialists and their disciplines. There was limited availability of printed journals, and there were high costs associated with each one. Imagine the work to print just one volume! Journal collections were based on what disciplines traditionally expected to have on hand as well as the consideration of the number of references appearing in journals per a designated time frame, known as the Gross and Gross method (Gross & Gross, 1927). Imagine, in the 1920s many chemistry journals had one article that had one reference while other articles had no references within a 5-year time frame. In other disciplines, such as physiology, the Gross and Gross method was found to be biased (Brodman, 1944). Per Brodman (1944), the Gross and Gross method was accepted because "any method was better than no method" (p. 482).

Let's fast-forward through time. Concepts of impact factor and citation indexing were first mentioned in a publication by Garfield (1955). The goals were to distinguish how the author's published works impacted the literature at large, create a trail of citations back to original works, and identify other authors' interests in similar topics. Hence the birth of the Science Citation Index in 1964 (Garfield, 2007). The index was originally developed to help publicize scientific literature and help researchers identify relevant literature.

Garfield and a colleague developed the Journal Impact Factor (JIF) to avoid the exclusion of relevant, smaller journals deemed important to the science discipline in the Science Citation Index (Garfield, 2007). The operational definition for JIF as reported by Garfield (1999) consists of a numerator and denominator. The numerator is the number of citations within the current year from all citable resources from the previous 2 years. The denominator is the number of published items (as specified) in the previous 2 years. Yes, it can be confusing, so here's an example.

We will explain JIF calculation using a hypothetical journal named *High Aspirations in Publishing*. In 2022, there were 548 citations made from all possible citable articles from the years 2020 and 2021 in that journal. In 2020, the journal published 88 citable articles, and 91 citable articles were published in 2021. The JIF is 548 / (88 + 91) = 548 / 179 = 3.06. The JIF for the hypothetical journal is 3. This is interpreted as each citable article published in 2020 and 2021 in that journal was cited at least three times.

The JIF is really about journal performance and not individual article performance. The JIF value indicates the journal has selected and published articles of value as reflected by these articles being cited in other journals. Journals with high JIF scores are usually prestigious and well-established journals.

As much as we want to measure our self-worth by publishing in prestigious journals, please avoid thinking your worth is tied to journal prestige! Excellent articles are submitted to prestigious journals all the time, and a large portion of excellent articles are rejected. Prestigious journals have a limited number of pages; therefore, a limited number of excellent articles are accepted per volume each year. If your manuscript is rejected, find another home after reviewing and considering the provided feedback from peer reviewers. Also consider that a skewed distribution in citations occurs in most science disciplines, which Garfield (2006) reports as a "20/80 phenomenon." The phenomenon is most citations (80%) stem from a few articles (20%). As published authors, we all want to claim that 20%.

Another metric is the Journal Citation Index (JCI), found in the annual Journal Citation Reports, which is a normed value that is easier to interpret and reflects how the level of journal impact and the value can be examined across journals from different disciplines (Clarivate, 2021). All journals have an average score of 1. If a journal has a score of 2, it is interpreted as being twice as impactful as compared to the average journal. If a journal has a JCI value of 0.5, the journal has an impact size half of the average journal.

There are some factors to consider if you want to count heavily on JIF and JCI to choose a journal to potentially publish your article. The higher the JIF and JCI, the more difficult it will be to publish your article, and the risk of rejection is high. Journal articles that are considered classics are not included in the calculation of JIF or JCI scores. Sometimes, cited content is inaccurate (which is why going back to the original source is crucial) or the cited source has nothing to do with the topic at hand. Determining what is a citable item and introducing it in the calculations can be a point of contention. Examples of points of contention may include commentaries, editorials, book reviews, and letters to the editor. Also, some JIF and JCI scores may be low because the journals are not the oldest journals in the discipline or may not have the same marketing resources.

Always include the mission of the journal, author instruction information, and the audience of the journal in making your selection along with the JIF and JCI scores. One area to note is that predatory journals may cite false JIF scores that cannot be found in reputable listings through Clarivate and Scopus. Predatory journals may report false JIF scores higher than prestigious, older journals.

Now that you know the background of JIF and understand JCI, consider the metrics as another tool to help choose a journal

## The "So What" Question About Predatory Journals

Journals that focus on money more than scholarship can be dangerous to both the body of knowledge for a discipline and to the career of an academic. Publications that don't have a rigorous peer review process often publish flawed research because there is either limited or no peer review. That's why you can submit a paper and have it accepted and published within a couple of weeks. One of the basic tenets of science is critical appraisal and review of the work. When that is lacking, it undermines science. When others cite flawed work and base further work on it, it damages the body of scientific work in the literature. Over the past decade, there's been an alarming growth of predatory journals. It's gotten more difficult to distinguish between reputable and predatory journals as the predatory journals have gotten so good at imitating reputable ones. When citations from predatory journals are used in reputable nursing journals, the potential to undermine and corrupt nursing science with noncredible information is alarming (Oermann et al., 2019). Promotion and tenure committees in colleges of nursing are strongly urged to develop policies addressing publication in predatory journals (Broome et al., 2021; Hulsey et al., 2023). Your reputation as a scholar and your promotion and tenure opportunities decline if you engage in predatory publishing. You can see why it's important to have guidance as you learn how to navigate the publishing landscape!

In addition to flawed science and author reputation, publishing in predatory journals can be expensive. Journal article processing charges range from a few hundred to a few thousand dollars. In many cases, it is impossible to get the payment refunded even after asking for a withdrawal of the article once the author realizes they made a mistake.

Is it possible to find good research in predatory journals? Of course it is, just as it is possible to have excellent faculty and courses in nonaccredited schools. But you'll be judged by the company you keep. And if you associate with predatory journals, everyone will figure that's the best company you could find. And of course, you're much better than that!

## Why Do Authors Continue Submitting to Predatory Journals?

Despite the problems related to predatory journals, there continue to be authors who submit their work to predatory journals. Kurt (2018) did a large study to determine why authors publish in predatory open-access journals. About 80% came from India, Pakistan, Turkey, China, the Philippines, Iran, Nigeria, Malaysia, Kenya, and Bangladesh. He identified four main categories of why authors published in predatory journals. One category that came up repeatedly was that researchers from developing countries felt they would be rejected by journals based in the Western world based on things such as lack of proficiency with the English language, having a Muslim last name and living in a Muslim country, or publishing research that is very specific to the country and might not be easily transferable to other settings. For these reasons, they felt more comfortable submitting to journals based out of their home countries, where many predatory journals are based.

The second category was a lack of awareness of the journal's reputation or even the whole idea of predatory journals. They were flattered to get an email inviting them, so they submitted a manuscript. Some universities did not consider it a problem to publish in these journals, so it was not considered a problem for the faculty member.

In addition, there is often pressure in academics to build up a curriculum vitae quickly in order to advance. Regular peer review can often spread out over 3 to 6 months, once revisions are made and reviewers evaluate the revisions. From original submission to publication can be a year to 15 months or longer. If you are trying to build your curriculum vitae quickly, the promise of quick review and publication is tempting.

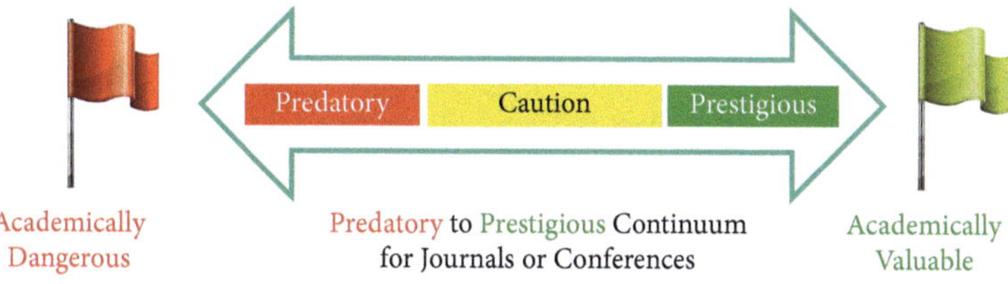



**FIGURE 5.1**  Predatory to prestigious continuum. (Copyright © 2012 Depositphotos/creatOR76.)

Now that you know what the problems are with predatory publications, and why authors persist despite the problems, let's look at some red flags that can help you initially assess a journal. Often the first contact may be that you get a strangely worded email invitation to submit your work. Commonly, the topic the sender is requesting has nothing to do with your expertise, but the sender claims to have found your prior work extremely valuable and impressive. The editorial board lists no nurses or even anyone with any expertise in anything remotely related to the journal title. When you don't reply, you receive follow-up emails that seem to border on harassment that ask you why you have not responded. Resist every urge to respond, as those are hallmark indicators of predatory journals.

Think of journals as creating a continuum ranging from extremely predatory (and academically dangerous) to prestigious (and academically valuable). Those that are reputable and highly respected are at one end of the continuum. Journals associated with established societies such as Sigma, the National League for Nursing, and American Association of Nurse Practitioners are examples of journals at the academically valuable end of the continuum (see Figure 5.1).

## "Open Access" Does Not Necessarily Mean "Predatory"

Don't be confused by reputable journals that meet quality criteria but use a fee-for-publication business model. The Directory of Open Access Journals is free and provides a list of open-access journals that meet standards for open access, journal website information, ISSN, quality control, licensing, and copyright. The advantage of this model is the material is available to a wider audience than subscription-based journals that are based on paying individually for the journal or paying professional association dues and receiving the journal as part of the membership. A great number of those who access academic journals do so through university library databases but must be affiliated with the university (as a faculty member or student) to gain access to the databases. Because Open Access is not limited to university library databases and does not depend on journal subscriptions, it allows much wider access than traditional business models. The cost can be high, however, ranging from a few hundred to a few thousand dollars.

Finding journals takes some investigation, but there are tools to help identify possible matches with reputable journals. A very helpful one is Journal /Author Name Estimator (JANE), a free online journal selection tool recommended for authors looking for health and biomedical journals. You can input keywords, a whole abstract, and other combinations of text to find recommendations of journals from PubMed/MEDLINE that would be a match. Another resource that provides an expansive list of journals is offered by Wiley. It allows you to review and compare journal metrics for up to four journals at a time. For a list of reputable nursing journals, the Nursing Journal Directory (n.d.) that has been vetted by the International Academy of Nursing Editors should be your go-to resource.

Colleague recommendations for publication possibilities are an important part of your search for a good match. You can add their experience with some of the journals to help determine whether you should submit to a specific journal.

## Manuscript Submission and Beyond

After following the author instructions of your carefully chosen journal, it's time to submit! Take a well-earned celebratory deep breath as you move into the next phase of publication. First, there's the waiting time. Depending on the journal, the time can vary from a few weeks to a few months. Much depends on the availability of reviewers and whether they are able to meet the expected deadline. And it will generally feel like the wait is far too long as you anxiously anticipate what you hope is a positive response from the journal's editor.

It is not impossible to have your manuscript accepted immediately and without any suggestions for revisions, but we have never actually met anyone this has happened to. It is more likely that you will receive peer reviewer feedback for revisions and an invitation to resubmit, or peer reviewer feedback and rejection of your manuscript in its current form.

What is important is that you try, try, and try again! Give yourself time to grapple with your emotions. Once you are ready, go back and read the feedback, which you may perceive differently after some time has passed. If you are invited to resubmit, by all means do so after addressing the reviewer comments.

If the decision is rejection, go back to the author worksheet and select one of the other journals. Before submitting the manuscript, make revisions using feedback from the journal peer reviewers. Integrating the feedback will make your manuscript stronger and decrease the possibility of another rejection.

Although you may want to discard or file the manuscript under "Haunted Manuscript," refrain from doing so. Manuscripts need to be rehomed. When ready to submit again, make sure to edit the cover letter. There are few journal management systems that have an item to report if the manuscript was previously submitted elsewhere and which journal. If the cover letter is not changed and the management system does not require you to report a previous submission, you have just outed yourself. Do not give the editor a reason to question your attention to detail. And of course, as with your initial submission, avoid the temptation to submit the manuscript to a predatory journal for all the reasons previously discussed. After all, your manuscript deserves better company than to possibly appear next to a hoax article like Baldassarre's (2020) "What's the Deal With Birds?"

# Reflection Exercises and Questions

1. Why it is important to disseminate the results of your project in reputable journals?

2. Fill out a publication worksheet and describe why you chose specific journals. Once you have three possible journals selected, use the Think, Check, Submit Checklist to review your choices.

Journals: Think. Check. Submit.

The checklist is a tool that will help you discover what you need to know when assessing whether or not a publisher is suitable for your research. The checklist is licensed under a Creative Commons Attribution 4.0 International License and reprinted here for your convenience.

How can you be sure the journal you are considering is the right journal for your research?

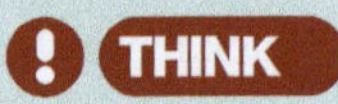


Are you submitting your research to a trusted journal?

Is it the right journal for your work?

- More research is being published worldwide.
- New publishers are launched each week.
- Many researchers have concerns about **predatory publishing**.
- It can be challenging to find up-to-date guidance when choosing where to publish.

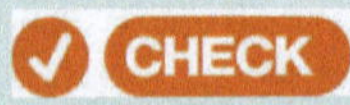


Reference this list for your chosen journal to check if it is trusted.

Do you or your colleagues know the journal?

Have you read any articles in the journal before?

Is it easy to discover the latest papers in the journal?

Name of the journal: the name is unique; it is not the same or easily confused with another journal.

Can you cross check with information about the journal in the **ISSN portal**?

## Can you easily identify and contact the publisher?

Is the publisher name clearly displayed on the journal website?

Can you contact the publisher by telephone, email, and post?

## Is the journal clear about the type of peer review it uses?

Does the website mention whether the process involves independent/external reviewers, how many reviewers per paper?

Is the publisher offering a review by an expert editorial board or by researchers in your subject area?

The journal doesn't guarantee acceptance or a very short peer review time.

## Are articles indexed and/or archived in dedicated services?

Will your work be indexed/archived in an easily discoverable database?

Does the publisher ensure **long-term archiving and preservation** of digital publications?

Does the publisher use permanent digital identifiers?

## Is it clear what fees will be charged?

Does the journal site explain what these fees are for and when they will be charged?

Does the publisher explain on their website how they are financially supported?

Do they mention the currency and amount of any fees?

Does the publisher website explain whether or not waivers are available?

**Are guidelines provided for authors on the publisher website?**

For open access journals, does the publisher have a clear <u>license</u> policy? Are there preferred licenses? Are there exceptions permitted depending on the needs of the author? Are license details included on all publications?

Does the publisher allow you to retain <u>**copyright**</u> of your work? Can you share your work via, for example, an institutional repository, and under what terms?

Does the publisher have a clear policy regarding potential conflicts of interest for authors, editors and reviewers?

Can you tell what formats your paper will be available in? (e.g. HTML, XML, PDF) Does the journal provide any information about <u>**metrics of usage or citations**</u>?

**Is the publisher a member of a recognized industry initiative?**

Are they a <u>**current member**</u> of the <u>**Committee on Publication Ethics (COPE)**</u> and follow its <u>**guidelines**</u>?

If the journal is open access, is it listed in the <u>**Directory of Open Access Journals (DOAJ)**</u>?

If the publisher offers an open access option, is it a <u>**current member**</u> of the <u>**Open Access Scholarly Publishers' Association (OASPA)**</u>?

Is the journal hosted on one of INASP's <u>**Journals Online**</u> platforms (for journals published in Bangladesh, Nepal, Sri Lanka, Central America, and Mongolia) or on <u>**African Journals Online**</u> (AJOL, for African journals)?

If the journal is open access, is it hosted on <u>**Scielo**</u> (for Latin American scientific journals)?

If the journal is open access, is it indexed in <u>**Latindex**</u> (for journals that are published in Latin America, the Caribbean, Spain, and Portugal)?

If the journal is open access, is it indexed by **Redalyc** (for journals that are published in Latin America and the Caribbean, Spain, and Portugal)?

Is the publisher a member of another trade association?

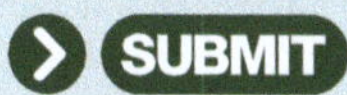


**If you have been able to check most or all of the items on the list.**
Complete the checklist and submit your manuscript only if you can answer "yes" to most or all of the questions above.



## Closing Scenario

"Drafting my publication worksheet was an eye-opening experience," Dr. Avila said thoughtfully. "It helped me decide in an intentional way what I was going to write about. I had started writing sections without the worksheet but realized it was very easy to get quickly unfocused. I like the one-sentence description because I know that if what I am writing about doesn't fit into that category, I'm not staying focused. At first, investigating journals was overwhelming, but with the guidelines about what to look for, the INANE list of vetted journals, the JANE name estimator, and the Think, Check, Submit list, I became more confident I could make a good journal choice. I also talked to some of the faculty who have published and found out about their experiences publishing in different journals. I've settled on one that I think best fits my manuscript."

"Sounds like you are ready to draft out that manuscript!" said Dr. Duran.

# References

American Psychological Association. (2020). *Publication manual of the American Psychological Association* (7th ed.). https://doi.org/10.1037/0000165-000

Baldassarre, D. T. (2020). What the deal with birds? *Scientific Journal of Research and Reviews, 2*(3). https://www.chm.bris.ac.uk/sillymolecules/birds.pdf

Brodman E. (1944). Choosing physiology journals. *Bulletin of the Medical Library Association, 32*(4), 479–483.

Broome, M. E., Oermann, M. H., Nicoll, L. H., Waldrop, J. B., Carter-Templeton, H., & Chinn, P. L. (2021). Publishing in predatory journals: Guidelines for nursing faculty in promotion and tenure policies. *Journal of Nursing Scholarship: An Official Publication of Sigma Theta Tau International Honor Society of Nursing, 53*(6), 746–752. https://doi.org/10.1111/jnu.12696

Clarivate. (2021). *Introducing the journal citation indicator: A new approach to measure the citation impact of journals in the Web of Science core collection.* https://clarivate.com/wp-content/uploads/dlm_uploads/2021/05/Journal-Citation-Indicator-discussion-paper.pdf

Committee on Publication Ethics. (2019). *Predatory publishing.* https://publicationethics.org/node/45216

Committee on Publication Ethics, Directory of Open Access Journals, Open Access Scholarly Publishers Association, & the World Association of Medical Editors. (2022). *Principles of transparency and best practice in scholarly publishing.* https://publicationethics.org/sites/default/files/principles-transparency-best-practice-scholarly-publishing.pdf

Conlogue, B. C., Gilman, N. V., & Holmes, L. M. (2022). Open access and predatory publishing: A survey of the publishing practices of academic pharmacists and nurses in the United States. *Journal of the Medical Library Association: JMLA, 110*(3), 294–305. https://doi.org/10.5195/jmla.2022.1377

Diers, D., & Downs, F. S. (1994). Colonizing: A measurement of the development of a profession. *Nursing Research, 43*(5), 316–318.

Garfield, E. (1955). Citation indexes for science: A new dimension in documentation through association of ideas. *Science, 122*(3159), 108–111. https://doi.org/10.1126/science.122.3159.108

Garfield E. (1999). Journal impact factor: A brief review. *CMAJ: Canadian Medical Association Journal, 161*(8), 979–980.

Garfield E. (2006). Commentary: Fifty years of citation indexing. *International Journal of Epidemiology, 35*, 1128. https://doi.org/10.1093/ije/dyl190

Garfield E. (2007). The evolution of the Science Citation Index. *International Microbiology: The Official Journal of the Spanish Society for Microbiology*, *10*(1), 65–69.

Gross, P. L. K., & Gross, E. M. (1927). College libraries and chemical education. *Science*, *66*(1713), 385–389. https://www.jstor.org/stable/1651803

Heinrich, K. T. (2008). *A nurse's guide to presenting and publishing: Dare to share.* Jones & Bartlett Learning.

Herrera, A., & Foronda, C. (2022). From bedside to webside: Telehealth education for doctoral nursing students. *Journal of Doctoral Nursing Practice*, *15*(3), 165–172. https://doi.org/10.1891/JDNP-2021-0049

Hulsey, T., Carpenter, R., Carter-Templeton, H., Oermann, M. H., Keener, T. A., & Maramba, P. (2023). Best practices in scholarly publishing for promotion or tenure: Avoiding predatory journals. *Journal of Professional Nursing: Official Journal of the American Association of Colleges of Nursing*, *45*, 60–63. https://doi.org/10.1016/j.profnurs.2023.01.002

Jamali, H. R., & Nikzad, M. (2011). Article title type and its relation with the number of downloads and citations. *Scientometrics*, *88*(2), 653–661. https://doi.org/10.1007/s11192-011-0412-z

Knudsen, S. V., Laursen, H. V. B., Johnsen, S. P., Bartels, P. D., Ehlers, L. H., & Mainz, J. (2019). Can quality improvement improve the quality of care? A systematic review of reported effects and methodological rigor in plan-do-study-act projects. *BMC Health Services Research*, *19*(1), 683. https://doi.org/10.1186/s12913-019-4482-6

Kurt, S. (2018). Why do authors publish in predatory journals? *Learned Publishing*, *31*(2), 141–147. https://doi.org/10.1002/leap.1150

Langford, C. A., & Pearce, P. F. (2019). Increasing visibility for your work: The importance of a well-written title. *Journal of the American Association of Nurse Practitioners*, *31*(4), 217–218. https://doi.org/10.1097/JXX.0000000000000212

Loyd, V., & Scaglione, K. (2022). Practicing upstream: Race-based trauma care training for veteran's health administration nurse practitioners. *Journal of Doctoral Nursing Practice*, *15*(3), 150–156. https://doi.org/10.1891/JDNP-2021-0013

McFarland, M.R., & Wehbe-Alamah, H.B. (2015). *Leininger's culture care diversity and universality: A worldwide nursing theory* (3rd ed.). Sudbury, MA: Jones and Bartlett Learning.

Merriam-Webster. (n.d.). *Slant.* https://www.merriam-webster.com/dictionary/slant

Monsivais, D. (2021). Is the title of your manuscript telling the truth? *Research and Theory for Nursing Practice: An International Journal*, *35*(2), 1–2.

Nursing Journal Directory (n.d.). https://airtable.com/app1QbygMN23wigqu/shrjqveaKHtS9xku8/tblNXTxmTr18CC1If

Oermann, M. H., Nicoll, L. H., Carter-Templeton, H., Woodward, A., Kidayi, P. L., Neal, L. B., Edie, A. H., Ashton, K. S., Chinn, P. L., & Amarasekara, S. (2019). Citations of articles in predatory nursing journals. *Nursing Outlook, 67*(6), 664–670. https://doi.org/10.1016/j.outlook.2019.05.001

Pearce, P. F., Hicks, R. W., & Pierson, C. A. (2018). Keywords matter: A critical factor in getting published work discovered. *Journal of the American Association of Nurse Practitioners, 30*(4), 179–181. https://doi.org/10.1097/JXX.0000000000000048

Pope, S., Rader, A., & Stansifer, S. (2022). Assessing vaccine hesitancy among pediatric healthcare providers. *Journal of Doctoral Nursing Practice, 15*(1), 65–71. https://doi.org/10.1891/JDNP-2021-0033

Rossi, M. J., & Brand, J. C. (2020). Journal article titles impact their citation rates. *Arthroscopy: The Journal of Arthroscopic & Related Surgery, 36*(7), 2025–2029. https://doi.org/10.1016/j.arthro.2020.02.018

Sword, H. (2012). *Stylish academic writing.* Harvard University Press.

Taylor, A. C., Hopkins, L. W., & Moore, G. (2021). Increasing human papillomavirus immunization in the primary care setting. *The Nurse Practitioner, 46*(10), 37–42. https://doi.org/10.1097/01.NPR.0000790528.06533.66

# Improving Authorship Skills Through Peer Reviewing

## Objectives

- Discuss the importance of manuscript peer review to the integrity of nursing scholarship.
- Identify resources for developing skills for manuscript peer review.
- Familiarize yourself with principles for promoting equity and social justice during the manuscript peer review process.

### Opening Scenario

Dr. Avila approaches her mentor and says, "After receiving the helpful review comments on my manuscript, I realized what an important role reviewers have. I want to find out how to become a reviewer, but it seems like a lot of work. Is it worth it?"

Dr. Duran says, "That's a question shared by many others. Think of it as a professional service like serving on committees or providing community service. And if there were no reviewers, when the time came for *your* manuscript to be reviewed, what would happen?"

Dr. Avila thoughtfully asks, "How do people learn how to be reviewers? Are there courses I can take or other resources to help me learn? What should I do to prepare?" Dr. Duran assures her she can provide professional development resources for peer reviewing and is also willing to provide mentorship in the process. Dr. Duran says she has always been committed to reviewing manuscripts as her own career was enhanced by those reviewers who took the time to provide constructive feedback delivered with kindness.

## Why Would Anyone Want to Be a Manuscript Peer Reviewer?

Before the availability of online manuscript submission services and other conveniences of the internet in general, journal editors would send out a manuscript to peer reviewers via regular mail. The reviewers would then write or type their comments and send them back to the editor by regular mail. As you can imagine, the time needed for this to occur was lengthy (3–4 months), even in the best of circumstances. Thankfully, online manuscript submission systems and the ability to provide reviewer feedback digitally have made the process much more efficient. In contrast to when we started peer reviewing, there are now peer review courses freely available from many publishers, making it much easier to gain foundational knowledge about the whole process. Without peer reviewing courses, learning best practices was trial and error. The type of feedback we received often helped shape our future feedback to others. If we received critical feedback without suggestions for improvement, we learned that we didn't want to be *that* kind of reviewer. If we received constructive feedback delivered with kindness, we learned how to provide helpful reviews and could pay it forward when providing feedback to others.

Even with online systems providing increased efficiency, there is no doubt that peer reviewing remains a time-intensive activity. So why should you spend hours working as a volunteer peer reviewer? Your time is precious, and you may think you cannot afford to spend time reviewing. Keep in mind reviewing is a service to the nursing profession at large. While less visible than providing community service through working at a health clinic or serving on a school committee, it is a critically important professional service. The peer review system is the quality assurance system that upholds the integrity of the discipline. Some consider it a professional responsibility (instead of just a "nice-to-do" service). They believe the responsibility was incurred when they were the beneficiaries of constructive reviews that ultimately helped them publish their manuscripts. They now "pay it forward" with the hope that others will do the same.

In addition to professional service, peer reviewing also provides fairly immediate benefits to you as a reviewer. You'll get a peek into the latest scholarly projects being done throughout the country. In addition, the review process will also help you improve your writing skills. When you identify problems with logic or flow in a manuscript, you are developing a skill that you can bring to your writing. However, it's no secret that it's always easier to identify problems when the work belongs to someone else! Being objective about your writing after investing so much effort into a manuscript can be almost impossible. That's why having colleagues who are willing to read and review your work before submitting it to a journal is so important.

Because reviewing lacks the visibility of working in a clinic or in-person committee work, it can easily fall into the "hidden work" category. Fortunately, there are mechanisms to provide recognition to reviewers. Some journals provide a certificate of appreciation at the end of each year recognizing the number of reviews that have been done. Another mechanism is the Web of Science Reviewer Recognition Services[T] (formerly Publons), which allows you to keep track of the number of papers you have reviewed for a journal and maintains reviewer anonymity. This type of recognition is helpful when you need to provide evidence of service for your professional portfolio. Many journal platforms are integrated with the Web of Science Reviewer Recognition service, and you can opt-in to receive credit when you submit your review.

## Becoming a Journal Peer Reviewer

There are many paths to becoming a reviewer. Start with your colleagues who already review for a specific journal that publishes articles that would fit your expertise. You can ask them to mentor you directly, and when you have developed the necessary skills, ask them to recommend you to the editor as a reviewer. The editor will almost certainly be delighted to add you to the peer reviewer pool. In addition to informal mentoring, there may be more structured mentorship programs available (Monsivais & Robbins, 2017). Professional societies and conferences also provide a chance to network with editors and members of the society, which may have their own journal. Some journals will issue a call for reviewers through editorials or social media, and you can reach out to the editor to let them know you are interested. The process is slightly different for each journal, ranging from an application process that requires that you submit a CV that is formally reviewed to a much more informal process such as simply volunteering.

As you look for reviewing opportunities, you can educate yourself through a variety of online resources. Here are a few of the many resources available to help develop skills as a peer reviewer. As reviewers are the gatekeepers to the publication world, they must be well educated about their role:

- Elsevier's Researcher Academy provides a Certified Peer Reviewer Course composed of 12 modules: https://researcheracademy.elsevier.com/navigating-peer-review/certified-peer-reviewer-course. If time is short, you may want to focus first on Module 3.1: "How to Write a Helpful Peer Review Report."

- Springer Nature provides tutorials on "How to Peer Review" that include quizzes to demonstrate competency: https://www.springernature.com/gp/authors/campaigns/how-to-peer-review

- Springer Publishing (a different group than Springer Nature) provides a helpful page of best practices and sample review comments: https://www.springerpub.com/journal-peer-reviewers

- Web of Science Academy-Clarivate™ provides free online modules about peer reviewing: https://clarivate.com/web-of-science-academy

- Wiley Author Services provides a detailed section about all aspects of peer reviewing: https://authorservices.wiley.com/Reviewers/journal-reviewers/indexhtml

While content expertise about a manuscript is definitely important, valuable reviewers also know the importance of deadlines and take their commitment to review by the deadline seriously. If they cannot finish a review on time, they notify the editor they will be delayed. They also commit to providing constructive, substantive feedback that will help improve the manuscript.

The Committee on Publication Ethics (2024) provides a detailed document outlining ethical guidelines for peer reviewers, which you may find helpful to download and keep available for reference. There are a few key points to keep in mind when you decide to accept a review invitation and register on the journal's site. First, provide accurate information when filling in the online reviewer information for the journal. Don't overstate your expertise in types of studies you are qualified to review, for example. This may lead to your receiving manuscripts that you simply don't have the background to review, which will not be able to be helpful to the author, the editor, or the state of the science. If you do receive a manuscript that is outside your scope of expertise, you may let the editor know that when you receive the review invitation. Second, competing interests fall into categories of personal, financial, intellectual, professional, political, or religious. There may be times you have a similar manuscript in preparation and you are simply curious about what is in the manuscript. That's a definite conflict, and curiosity is not a reason to agree to review a manuscript. If there might be a reason you would be biased for or against a certain topic, you would want to notify the editor and decline the review assignment. Third, you'll need to make the time in your calendar to "find" it. Let's face it, blocks of time don't just magically appear when something needs to be done. Accepting a review assignment comes with the obligation to schedule time to do the work. It will always take at least twice as long as you think it will to do a careful review. Often reviewers may spend 2 to 4 hours providing feedback on a manuscript. Schedule it on your calendar just as you would other commitments. Generally, a few short sessions are more realistic and allow a more comprehensive review than one long session. Second and third readings of the manuscript usually allow a more in-depth perspective and enhanced understanding of the work.

## Reviewing DNP Quality Improvement Manuscripts Versus Research-Focused Manuscripts

Resources for reviewers often focus on primary research, but the focus of DNP-related projects is usually practice oriented with the aim of improving patient outcomes. DNP projects generally use quality improvement or evidence-based practice frameworks, so the purpose and focus are different than primary research. Reporting guidelines will generally be aligned with the Standards for Quality Improvement Reporting Excellence (SQUIRE 2.0).

## Promoting Equity and Social Justice

In addition to reporting guidelines, there are other areas to consider when reviewing. Our implicit biases are those automatic reactions that are outside of our conscious control. Automatic reactions we have toward certain groups of people or situations may impact the review we provide, so becoming aware of our own biases is important so that we don't perpetuate biases in the literature. Reduction of biases in practice and scholarship are included in the American Association of Colleges of Nursing (AACN, 2021) Essentials 3.2e: "Challenge biases and barriers that impact population health outcomes."

Bias is defined as "the action of supporting or opposing a particular person or thing in an unfair way, because of allowing personal opinions to influence your judgment" (Cambridge Dictionary, n.d.). In the case of a manuscript review, reviewers may have strong opinions on an almost unlimited variety of topics.

Fitzgerald and Hurst (2017) found ample evidence that healthcare professionals demonstrate implicit biases at a similar degree as the general population. With a focus specifically on nursing, both Narayan (2019) and Wei et al. (2023) found implicit biases demonstrated for race/ethnicity, sexuality, age, physical and mental health conditions, and substance abuse disorders. Implicit biases can perpetuate healthcare disparities, and recognizing one's own biases is an important first step toward promoting a more equitable environment.

A comprehensive starting point is Project Implicit (2011), a network of researchers investigating thoughts and feelings outside of conscious awareness and control. There are a variety of implicit bias tests for age, weight, disability, transgender, religion, race, and many more. Watch "Implicit Bias" (McCombs School of Business, 2019) and consider what biases are part of your worldview. Did you have any "aha" moments?

Along with self-awareness of one's own biases, reviewers also must be aware of principles for actively reducing bias as they review. The American Psychological Association (2020) provides general guidelines for reducing bias for authors and reviewers. The guidelines include focusing on relevant participant characteristics for the project, acknowledging relevant differences do exist in relation to the target population, being appropriately specific (about age, health condition, socioeconomic status, gender identity, disability, etc.), acknowledging people's humanity, providing operational definitions and labels, and providing parallel designation for groups such as racial and ethnic identity information. Buchanan et al. (2021) provide an excellent discussion and illuminating examples.

The following table is a peer-reviewer guide that incorporates general review suggestions based on SQUIRE guidelines and COPE (and other sources,) along with suggested areas for review based on Fallon et al. (2022) if the manuscript deals with social justice issues. We have also included sample comments that are constructive and sample comments that are *not* constructive in the last two columns.

**TABLE 6.1** Peer Reviewer Guide

| Section | General Review SQUIRE Criteria, COPE, and Other Sources for Reviewers | If the Topic Is Relevant to Social Justice/Marginalized Groups Fallon et al. (2022) | Sample Constructive Comments | Sample Nonconstructive Comments |
|---|---|---|---|---|
| Prereview | Consider<br>• your expertise with the content, methods<br>• time commitment needed<br>• any conflicts of interest | Consider<br>• your position in relation to the content<br>• your personal assumptions<br>• your background in structural racism and health research/ familiarity with antiracist principles | Positionality statement helps understand the author's commitment to the purpose of the project and point of view. | Not sure why the "statement" is included. Is this necessary? |
| Title | Does it reflect an initiative to improve health care? (quality, safety, effectiveness, patient centeredness, timeliness, cost, efficiency, and equity of health care, or access to it)<br><br>Does the title match the manuscript's content? | | The title should contain keywords such as *quality, safety, effectiveness, patient centeredness, timeliness, cost efficiency,* and *equity of health care,* or access to it.<br><br>Keywords important for assigning correct MeSH headings. | I am confused by the title. |
| Topic | Relevant and timely topic?<br>Within the scope of the journal?<br>Interesting to readers? | | Stronger emphasis on why prior attempts to correct this longstanding problem have not been successful. | References outdated. |
| Abstract | Relevant keywords are included. Information is summarized using abstract format of the journal. | Conveys system-centered language instead of deficit-oriented language | Keywords and phrases are not evident in the abstract. Important for assigning MeSH headings. | Needs additional information. |
| Introduction | | | | |
| Problem Description | Nature and significance of the local problem | | | |

| Section | General Review SQUIRE Criteria, COPE, and Other Sources for Reviewers | If the Topic Is Relevant to Social Justice/Marginalized Groups Fallon et al. (2022) | Sample Constructive Comments | Sample Nonconstructive Comments |
|---|---|---|---|---|
| Available Knowledge | Summary of what is known about the problem, including relevant previous studies and quality gap or knowledge gap at local level<br><br>Integrated synopsis versus listing of individual studies | The review draws from a broad historical, and cultural base.<br><br>Do participant samples reflect the diversity of the population of interest?<br><br>How do studies in review report race, ethnicity, gender identity, and so forth?<br><br>How do studies reviewed consider heterogeneity in marginalized populations?<br><br>Stigmatizing terms avoided. | It would be helpful to the reader to point out how earlier studies do not emphasize inequities in the system (structural racism) and how the inequities are tied to health outcomes. | Do not think including comments about marginalized groups or social justice is helpful to the study. |
| Rationale | Rationale = Reasons authors have for expecting the intervention will work<br><br>Could be a formal theory or informal framework, models, and concepts, to explain the problem, any reasons or assumptions that were used to develop the intervention(s), and reasons the intervention(s) was expected to work | Does the theoretical lens center on the perspectives of marginalized groups? (Or are the perspectives of privileged groups reinforced?)<br><br>Does the theoretical lens match the methods? | Expanding description of the theory used would help the reader better understand the perspective of the target population. | Not sure space should be used for theory background. Do not see how it has relevance to the study. |

(continued)

**TABLE 6.1** (continued)

| Section | General Review SQUIRE Criteria, COPE, and Other Sources for Reviewers | If the Topic Is Relevant to Social Justice/Marginalized Groups Fallon et al. (2022) | Sample Constructive Comments | Sample Nonconstructive Comments |
|---|---|---|---|---|
| Specific Aims | Aims should align with the problem significance and gap identified in the introduction and reflect the rationale for the project. If appropriate, aims state how both process and outcomes will be assessed. | Aims tied to an identified gap | A clearer link of aims to the problem statement would be helpful. | Do not see why this topic is needed to start with. |
| Methods | | | | |
| Context | Contextual elements (location, patient population, size, staffing, practice type, etc.) are considered important at the outset of introducing the intervention(s). | Author positionality statement to help readers better understand the connection to the topic Do authors consider heterogeneity in marginalized population? How are data on cultural identity reported (race, ethnicity, gender)? | Greater emphasis on contextual factors such as setting and team would help reader understand if the project would be useful in their own setting. | Provide more background . |
| Intervention(s) | Sufficient details were provided so others could reproduce it. Specifics about the team are involved. | | Would be helpful to include more specifics about the characteristics of the team that conducted the intervention. | Who was involved? |
| Study of the Intervention | Approach for assessing the impact of the intervention Approach used to find out if outcomes were due to the intervention | | A clearer description of how the outcome was assessed (e.g., surveys to find out if patients used the material). | Cannot tell how outcome was assessed. |

| Section | General Review SQUIRE Criteria, COPE, and Other Sources for Reviewers | If the Topic Is Relevant to Social Justice/Marginalized Groups Fallon et al. (2022) | Sample Constructive Comments | Sample Nonconstructive Comments |
| --- | --- | --- | --- | --- |
| Measures/ Instruments | Rationale for choosing measures and their operational definitions | Do the authors use culturally sensitive approaches in measuring constructs? | Explain validity and reliability of the measures to help readers better assess outcomes. | Missing information about measures. |
| Analysis | Qualitative and quantitative methods are used to draw inferences from the data. | | Would benefit from more detail so replication is possible. | Unable to tell how data were analyzed. |
| Ethical Considerations | IRB/potential COI | | Please describe how potential ethical concerns were reviewed and addressed. | IRB? |
| Results | a. initial steps of the intervention(s) and their evolution over time (e.g., timeline diagram, flow chart, or table), including modifications made to the intervention during the project<br>b. details of the process measures and outcome<br>c. contextual elements that interacted with the intervention(s)<br>d. observed associations between outcomes, interventions, and relevant contextual elements<br>e. unintended consequences such as unexpected benefits, problems, failures, or costs associated with the intervention(s).<br>Details about missing data | If structural variables create a disadvantage, do authors challenge mainstream values or theories to the sample in question? | Structural variables such as the organization and location, payer mix, practice type, leadership motivation, and numerous other factors will impact outcomes. Please address these variables. | Need more detail. |

(continued)

**TABLE 6.1**  (*continued*)

| Section | General Review SQUIRE Criteria, COPE, and Other Sources for Reviewers | If the Topic Is Relevant to Social Justice/Marginalized Groups Fallon et al. (2022) | Sample Constructive Comments | Sample Nonconstructive Comments |
|---|---|---|---|---|
| Discussion | | | | |
| Summary | Key findings, including relevance to the rationale and specific aims<br><br>Particular strengths of the project | | Please link findings back to the significance and aims of the project. | Summary needs improvement. |
| Interpretation | a. Nature of the association between the intervention(s) and the outcomes<br>b. Comparison of results with findings from other publications<br>c. Impact of the project on people and systems<br>d. Reasons for any differences between observed and anticipated outcomes, including the influence of context<br>e. Costs and strategic trade-offs, including opportunity costs | Recognition of structural factors that cause inequities<br><br>Implications for practice that have the potential to advance social justice | Do you have any insights on what the most important factors were in the outcomes? Or alternative explanations for the outcomes? | Outcomes are too simplistic and need detail. |
| Limitations | Factors that may have limited internal validity such as design imprecision<br>Factors that limit transferability | | More details will help readers assess results/identify factors that would influence future studies. | Limitations?? |

| Section | General Review SQUIRE Criteria, COPE, and Other Sources for Reviewers | If the Topic Is Relevant to Social Justice/Marginalized Groups Fallon et al. (2022) | Sample Constructive Comments | Sample Nonconstructive Comments |
| --- | --- | --- | --- | --- |
| Conclusions | a. Usefulness of the work<br>b. Sustainability<br>c. Potential for spread to other contexts<br>d. Implications for practice and for further study in the field<br><br>Suggested next steps | | Conclusions are appropriately related to findings. Would revise wording to say the intervention has the *potential* to improve practice instead of *will* improve practice. | Overstated conclusion. |
| Funding | Described in detail | | Important to mention funding so readers can assess whether funding may have influenced outcomes. | Funding? |
| Idea Development | | | | |
| Organized, Clear, Effective Transitions | CUNY assessment test in writing rubric sections | | | |
| Sentences and Word Choice Effectively Convey Ideas | | | The content is important and would be more clearly conveyed if sentence structure was simplified in some areas. | The authors need help with English language |
| Grammar, Usage, and Mechanics | | | Professional editing for writing mechanics would help the reader grasp the important content. | Many areas where meaning is not clear. |

## Closing Scenario

After following up on Dr. Duran's professional development recommendations, Dr. Avila enthusiastically tells Dr. Duran she's completed the Certified Peer Reviewer Course and has volunteered to be a journal peer reviewer with a journal she reads regularly. The editor has promised to send out a review invitation as soon as a manuscript that matches her expertise is submitted. Dr. Avila (looking a little embarrassed) shares with Dr. Duran that she took some of the tests in Project Implicit and was surprised to find out she carries an ageist bias in addition to biases against certain health conditions. Dr. Duran reminds her of the research showing nurses are not immune to bias, as biases are part of being human, and the key is recognizing one's own biases and taking action to not let them interfere with practice, scholarship, or service. Emily expresses appreciation for Dr. Duran's guidance in becoming a peer reviewer and acknowledges the important role peer review has in the integrity of nursing scholarship.

## Application Exercises

1. What types of biases did you discover you held through taking some of the Project Implicit tests?

2. Exchange manuscript drafts with a colleague and use the peer reviewer table to provide feedback to each other.

3. Springer Nature has quizzes that go with their modules: https://www.onlineexambuilder.com/how-to-peer-review/exam-87197?PHPSESSID=new. Take one!

## References

American Association of Colleges of Nursing. (2021). The essentials: Core competencies for professional nursing education. https://www.aacnnursing.org/Portals/42/AcademicNursing/pdf/Essentials-2021.pdf

American Psychological Association. (2020). *Publication manual of the American Psychological Association* (7th ed.). https://doi.org/10.1037/0000165-000

Buchanan, N. T., Perez, M., Prinstein, M. J., & Thurston, I. B. (2021). Upending racism in psychological science: Strategies to change how science is conducted, reported, reviewed, and disseminated. *The American Psychologist*, 76(7), 1097–1112. https://doi.org/10.1037/amp0000905

Cambridge Dictionary. (n.d.). *Bias*. https://dictionary.cambridge.org/us/dictionary/english/bias#google_vignette

Committee on Publication Ethics (2024). *Ethical guidelines for peer reviewers, COPE guidance*. https://publicationethics.org/resources/guidelines/cope-ethical-guidelines-peer-reviewers

Fallon, L., Grapin, S., Newman, D. S., & Noltemeyer, A. (2022). Promoting equity and social justice in the peer review process: Tips for reviewers. *School Psychology International*, 43(1), 12–17. https://doi-org.utep.idm.oclc.org/10.1177/01430343211070165

Fitzgerald, C., & Hurst, S. (2017). Implicit bias in healthcare professionals: a systematic review. *BMC Medical Ethics*, 18(19). https://doi.org/10.1186/s12910-017-0179-8

McCombs School of Business. (2019). *Implicit bias | Concepts unwrapped* [Video]. YouTube. https://www.youtube.com/watch?v=OoBvzI-YZf4

Monsivais, D., & Robbins, L. K. (2017). Mentoring the next generation of peer reviewers: A triple win. *The Canadian Journal of Nursing Research = Revue canadienne de recherche en sciences infirmieres*, 49(4), 139–141. https://doi.org/10.1177/0844562117739769

Narayan, M. C. (2019). CE: Addressing implicit bias in nursing: A review. *The American Journal of Nursing*, 119(7), 36–43. https://doi.org/10.1097/01.NAJ.0000569340.27659.5a

Project Implicit (2011). https://implicit.harvard.edu/implicit/takeatest.html

Wei, H., Price, Z., Evans, K., Haberstroh, A., Hines-Martin, V., & Harrington, C. C. (2023). The state of the science of nurses' implicit bias: A call to go beyond the face of the other and revisit the ethics of belonging and power. *Advances in Nursing Science*, 46(2), 121–136. https://doi.org/10.1097/ANS.0000000000000470

# The Future of Scholarly Communication in Nursing

## Objectives

- Become familiar with future trends in scholarly communication in nursing.
- Develop an appreciation for future-oriented skills needed as an academic author.
- Recognize ethical responsibilities related to the use of artificial intelligence.

## Opening Scenario

Dr. Avila lets her mentor know that she's just completed her first manuscript review for a journal and that she is confident the review comments will make the paper stronger. She continues by saying, "I found that by having the sample constructive comments available, I was easily able to focus on each section and see what needed to be done. I also realized my own manuscripts will be improved now that I have started being a reviewer. I know there are so many changes happening in authorship and publishing right now, and I'm wondering what kind of things I need to do to prepare."

Dr. Duran says, "While it's hard to know exactly what will happen, there are some trends that we can follow. First, let's look at what will remain the same. Skills such as critical appraisal of the literature, identifying knowledge gaps, and use of a particular theory to tie the work into what has already been done will continue to need the author's critical thinking skills. In some cases, AI may be able to make the initial investigation on some of those processes a little quicker, but it cannot critically think and place information in context. Fortunately, a knowledgeable human is still needed for that part!

"And for aspiring and established authors, the need to stay emotionally fit for scholarly work will remain unchanged. Those behavioral (making time and space for writing), artisanal (ongoing skill development), social (interaction and feedback with others), and emotional habits (thinking that emphasizes pleasure and growth) (Sword, 2017) that best support our writing will remain critical to success. The need for careful planning for all phases of writing either as a solo author or with others (coauthorship) also will not change. The critical thinking skills, behaviors, and relational skills needed for successful authorship will always be extremely important, and you've done a great job of starting to develop them. As you develop further as an author, you'll continually add new skills. Although some of the newer skills needed for authorship may have a learning curve attached, they are more concrete and task oriented than critical thinking or relational skills. Skills such as creating infographics, writing for varied audiences, and using AI to be more efficient all have a variety of professional development opportunities available." Dr. Avila looks intrigued and says she is anxious to start learning more about those skills.

# Traditional Scholarly Publishing

The traditional academic publishing model has long faced many challenges, and the rapid changes occurring will help alleviate some of the challenges. The challenges listed here are drawn from a variety of sources and the authors' own experiences.

One major challenge is the expense of the traditional print publishing model. In addition, there are often space limitations due to the expense of printing, which means some important research can face potential delays in dissemination. Printing also has a potential environmental impact, and publishers are now moving to more sustainable models of printing such as recycled paper and digital printing. Additionally, many publishers have gone to an online-only journal, which produces less of an environmental footprint.

Another challenge with the traditional publishing model is the lack of access to some academic journals. Access to academic journals is often limited unless you can use a university library, have a subscription to the journal, or are willing to pay the one-time access fee (generally $35–$45). In recent years many university libraries have had to discontinue some subscription services because of budget constraints, limiting access even further. And access becomes even more limited because of copyright restrictions. When authors assign copyright to the publisher, authors may not be able to share their work in open access areas such as university repositories.

The slow pace of the traditional publishing model poses another challenge. There is often a 1-to-2-year lag from submission to publication due to the length of time for reviews and revisions. If the journal publication schedule is three or four times a year, then dissemination can potentially be delayed due to publication scheduling. The slow pace built into the traditional model delays the availability of scholarly findings for others to use. Additionally, as discussed in Chapter 6, the traditional model of peer review is generally not transparent and can easily include bias. Biased peer review may eliminate some research that is worthy of publication, thereby making it unavailable to other scholars who would benefit from knowing the findings. The multiple challenges of expense, limited access, slow dissemination time, and potential for bias in peer review have led to alternatives to the traditional publishing model.

## Alternatives to Traditional Scholarly Publishing

Fortunately, there are newer dissemination models that provide wider access to scholarly findings than the traditional publishing model. Reputable open access journals (that were introduced in Chapter 5) are one popular solution. The research becomes available to readers at no cost, but the author or the author's funding agency pays to make the article open access. *Nursing Open*

(Wiley) is one example of an open access journal specifically for the nursing discipline.

Another popular dissemination model is preprint servers. A preprint is a finished manuscript posted to a server by the author before peer review or being published in a journal. Preprints serve the purposes of receiving feedback before submission to a journal, documenting the date a discovery or treatment was reported, and rapid dissemination. Despite the obvious benefits, there are also drawbacks to preprints. Drawbacks include the possibility of misinformation in the manuscript since it hasn't been peer reviewed, difficulty finding the preprint as it is not indexed on PubMed, and journal policies about preprints that restrict future publication in the journal (Flanagin et al., 2020; Oermann & Nicoll, 2020).

Watson (2020) provides an overview of three preprint servers that may be most useful for nursing, along with directions for using them: medRxiv, Authorea, and WikiJournal of Medicine. Before posting a preprint, it is important to consider the ramifications of doing so, and Castner et al. (2020) provide guiding questions to help make the decision.

Platforms such as Academia.edu and ResearchGate are academic social networks that can widen the visibility of your work and increase opportunities for collaboration. A word of caution about copyright: It is important to make sure you have permission from the publisher to publicly share your work. For example, Springer (2023) has policies about self-archiving and sharing.

Institutional repositories are another mechanism for sharing the work of researchers from the institution by making the work easily accessible for anyone who wishes to use them. The benefits to the researcher include a place to archive and manage all scholarly work in the same place so that the work gets maximum visibility.

## Academic Authorship Skills for the Future

As an author, the skills you will need for the future may look a little different than the ones you need right now. Yarris et al. (2020)

provide an excellent overview of the trends for authors that are becoming more evident. Some of these trends include more dynamic content (e.g., audio and visual content) replacing text, podcasts, and blogs commonly seen as supplemental resources to an article, curated content replacing primary literature, global knowledge sharing increasing as collaborative writing increases, and increasing the use of artificial intelligence (AI). We'll delve more deeply into these in the next section.

## Dynamic Content Instead of Text Content

Visual abstracts present your key points in images or graphics in a more engaging way than simply using text. They help the reader find the content most relevant to them to decide if they want to read the whole article. Visual abstracts (see Figure 7.1) work well on social media to disseminate the work to a wider audience than the author would have solely in the journal, which may have limited access for a majority of those who would be interested (Millar & Lim, 2022; Spicer & Coleman, 2022; Traboco et al., 2022). In addition to the scholarship underpinning visual abstracts, the references also contain a "how-to" component as well as helpful examples.

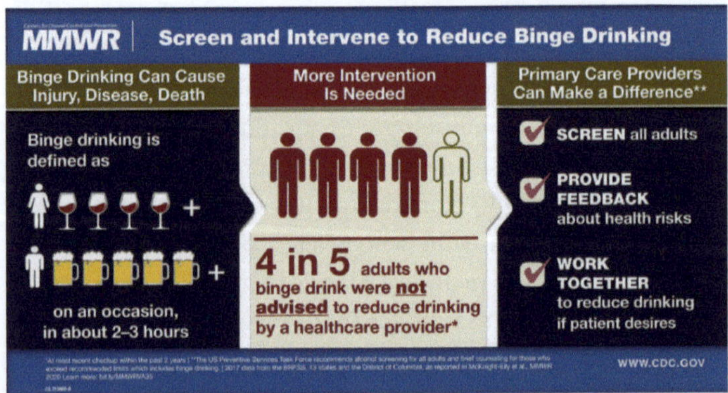


**FIGURE 7.1** Example of a visual abstract. (Source: Centers for Disease Control and Prevention, "Screen and Intervene to Reduce Binge Drinking," https://www.cdc.gov/ncbddd/fasd/screen-and-intervene-to-reduce-binge-drinking.html.)

If you would like to expand your reading even further, numerous sites can help you develop or provide examples of a visual abstract:

- https://www.myamericannurse.com/visual-abstracts-maximize-interest-and-impact/
- https://guides.mclibrary.duke.edu/gettingpublished/visualabstracts
- https://www.nursing.upenn.edu/academics/doctor-of-nursing-practice-dnp/dnp-scholarly-projects/

## Supplemental Resources to Published Articles

Supplemental resources (e.g., podcasts and blogs) for published articles are becoming increasingly available. Podcasts can offer additional insights from the author about the article, such as why the author became interested in the topic. The supplementary information can help readers deepen their understanding of the content.

## Curated Content

*Curated is* defined as "carefully chosen and thoughtfully organized and presented" (Merriam-Webster, n.d.). Content curation entails collecting, processing, and communicating information (Mullins, 2023) either for patients or colleagues. As the volume of medical literature on a topic often makes reading all individual articles impossible, those who can curate content will possess a valuable skill.

## Collaboration

Collaborative writing projects are trending in nursing and the health sciences, which increases the diversity of perspectives offered to readers as well as a shared workload. A collaborative approach to publishing a DNP project may involve colleagues, community stakeholders, and even patients in the project. But as with any group endeavor, conflict can easily arise. Collaboration increases the need for meticulous planning and authoring agreements like those that are available in Chapter 3. With plans in place and open and honest discussion before the project begins, the project will have the highest chances of success. There are a variety of collaboration tools, such as shared online workspaces and reference management systems, to enhance the efficiency and productivity of the team (Hermanns & Parker, 2020).

Collaboration can also help with creating a writing habit, which can be very difficult. There are always plenty of reasons not to get started writing, or if you get started, not to follow through. Whether you're in academics or practice, the competing demands for your time and attention can easily displace the time you have set aside to work on a manuscript.

Fortunately, there are strategies to help you make writing more of a habit and less of a "when I have time" idea. The Writing Accountability Group (WAG) model (Johns Hopkins Medicine, 2024) has a track record of success, and the time demands are minimal. WAGs emphasize the *process* of a writing habit and meet once a week for an hour over 10 weeks. No more than eight people are in a group, and writing (or a manuscript-related activity such as working on a data table) is done individually for 30 minutes during weekly 1-hour sessions. The first 15 minutes are allocated for reporting the previous week's progress and stating goals for the current session. The final 15 minutes are for the members to report whether they met their goal for the session and state their goal for the upcoming week (e.g., writing for 20 minutes per day). All the information related to this model is available on the Johns Hopkins site, including a WAG toolkit and podcasts for learning more about them.

Our own experiences with participating in a WAG group reinforce the benefits. We would like to emphasize the importance of having participants commit to being able to attend scheduled sessions and staying on track during reporting. The tendency is for other participants to start offering advice if someone needs assistance, and the report can quickly go into overtime. To keep the session on time, our solution was to allow those who wished to stay after the scheduled session the opportunity to give or seek advice from peers.

## Artificial Intelligence

AI offers great potential for helping authors increase efficiency. Tasks such as drafting an outline to help list ideas and structure content are ways that AI may increase efficiency by saving you the time of putting the information together from multiple sources. If it's not quite what you want, you can ask your AI platform (e.g., ChatGPT) for refinements in output by providing it with another prompt. But be careful! Since an AI platform draws from a large number of online resources, it may put ideas together that create erroneous links between ideas and create references that don't exist (known as "hallucinating"). If you are familiar with the content area, it will probably be easy to spot incorrect information, erroneous links, or an illogical flow of ideas. However, if all the information is new, it stands to reason you won't be able to do that. But whether the content is familiar or new, you'll need to closely fact-check both the text and any references included. In some cases, such as summarizing ideas and synthesizing information, it may take as long (or even longer) to use AI because of the need to carefully check all the details. Chasing down and identifying incorrect references or erroneous links between ideas usually takes longer than locating valid references and using your own critical thinking skills to synthesize the content.

Editing and proofreading using AI editing tools is a great way to identify typos, punctuation errors, and multiple grammar problems. Grammarly is one example, and Microsoft Word includes spelling and grammar checks. Here's a simple example of why fact-checking and knowledge as a content expert need to be used in conjunction with AI tools: Some grammar and spell-checking software may not recognize medical terminology and will flag areas that are not really errors. Your knowledge as a content expert in addition to your ability to fact-check is necessary to override the flagged medical terms that are actually correct.

For those who like to capture ideas by dictation, AI tools are available on a smartphone or computer. The ability to quickly dictate a Word document is now easily accomplished with the "Dictate" icon in Microsoft Word. AI can also generate images. Reed (2023) provides examples of AI tools that generate images of complex ideas that help students understand ideas more fully by supporting visual learning.

## Ethics Related to AI

AI brings with it both exciting possibilities and genuine concerns. Concerns related to ethics, legal issues, risk of bias, plagiarism, and misinformation in content and citations are some of the major concerns identified in a systematic review by Sallam (2023). When considering AI, authorship ethics take on a new layer of complexity.

The International Committee of Medical Journal Editors (2022) states the author is responsible for the integrity of the work. That includes accurate content, accurate references, acknowledging writing assistance with AI or a medical writer, and challenging biases that are built into the system under discussion. Authors are responsible for the accuracy of the content, including citations that accurately support the information in the manuscript. If the author does not carefully read the primary source, misinterpreting it can easily occur. Or, if AI is used, nonexistent citations may be generated. This is not only a problem for the reader of the individual article, but with citation error rates in various scientific disciplines ranging from 25%–54% (Rivkin, 2020), the nonexistent citation problem will compound the error rate greatly.

As biases are frequently part of the current literature, AI may easily incorporate them into suggested writing. AI-generated texts can be reviewed using the peer reviewer table from Chapter 6, which incorporates suggestions by Fallon et al. (2022) to recognize biases.

## Acknowledging AI Writing Assistance

Here are recommendations from the International Committee of Medical Journal Editors (2022):

> At submission, the journal should require authors to disclose whether they used artificial intelligence (AI)-assisted technologies (such as Large Language Models [LLMs], chatbots, or image creators) in the production

of submitted work. Authors who use such technology should describe, in both the cover letter and the submitted work, how they used it. Chatbots (such as ChatGPT) should not be listed as authors because they cannot be responsible for the accuracy, integrity, and originality of the work, and these responsibilities are required for authorship (see Section II.A.1). Therefore, humans are responsible for any submitted material that included the use of AI-assisted technologies. Authors should carefully review and edit the result because AI can generate authoritative-sounding output that can be incorrect, incomplete, or biased. Authors should not list AI and AI-assisted technologies as an author or co-author, nor cite AI as an author. Authors should be able to assert that there is no plagiarism in their paper, including in text and images produced by the AI. Humans must ensure there is appropriate attribution of all quoted material, including full citations. (Section 4).

Remember, AI is an adjunct tool, and your expertise and critical thinking must be part of the process to ensure the accuracy and logical consistency of the content.

## Reflection Questions

1.  What skills do I want to develop that will help me be a competitive academic author going forward?

2.  Which of your colleagues might be willing to form a WAG group with you?

## Application Exercises

1.  Create a visual abstract of your DNP project and share it with a colleague.

2.  After listening to any podcasts that supplement journal articles, create a podcast by having a colleague interview you about your project.

## Closing Scenario

Dr. Avila meets with Dr. Duran and says, "I'm excited about the possibilities in the future of scholarly communication. I can't wait to try a visual abstract and ask AI to brainstorm ideas with me! I've been thinking back to when we first started meeting and realized how far I've come with your mentorship. I retook the writing self-efficacy assessment that I did when we first started working together and found I scored much higher than I did when I first took it. I appreciate all feedback on my writing at a much deeper level and found my ability to discern what feedback should be incorporated has become much better. I've become much more skilled at synthesizing information and finding the literature gaps. And I think I've been developing my writing voice, which has been exciting for me. Writing is also now an activity that is on my calendar on a regular basis, and I am starting to feel as though something is missing if I am not writing a little almost every day.

"The WAG group I formed with three of my colleagues has been a great source in helping to develop everyone's writing habits, and after our 1 hour each week, we often get together for lunch and brainstorm new ideas and just socialize. They've become my friends as well as colleagues. In fact, two of us found a topic of mutual interest and will coauthor it. Of course, we'll develop an authorship agreement first and then develop a publication worksheet and investigate possible journals for submission. Even though I'm still a novice, I'm feeling much more confident about myself as an academic author!"

## Book Wrap-Up

Publishing DNP project outcomes is more critical than ever. Our rapidly changing and chaotic health care system is urgently in need of practical solutions, and translational research published by DNP scholars can play a large role in providing those solutions. Unfortunately, the challenges in academic writing can be overwhelming. There is so much to know in addition to sentence structure and grammar rules! Understanding and applying middle-range nursing-focused theories to clinical situations; the ability to make a place for your work in the literature; applying EBP, QI, and change frameworks; and using reporting guidelines are all foundational to manuscript development in the discipline of nursing. And foundational knowledge is just the beginning. We've considered the importance of being aware and in control of your emotions about writing. Everyone has a list of frustrations related to writing, and those lists are usually long. But once you normalize them as part of the process, and not a sign that you shouldn't be writing, your emotional fitness for writing improves. Developing habits such as scheduling writing time on your calendar and carrying out behaviors that support your physical and emotional health also play a critical role in writing success.

Transforming a DNP project report into a manuscript generally takes a lot of work and guidance from an experienced published author, who may be a potential coauthor. When you reach out to others (or others reach out to you) to coauthor a manuscript, it is important to know the benefits and challenges of coauthorship. There are resources such as authorship grids, partnership agreements, writing agreements, and colleague support agreements to mitigate some of the challenges.

Interestingly, the skills you develop as a manuscript peer reviewer will benefit your own writing (as well as provide a valuable service to the profession), so investing the time and energy in professional development is well worth it. There are many free, online resources available. And, although some technical skills for publishing may look a little different in the future, the good news is resources are available right now to help you start learning. The other good news is that the essential writing skills, such as critical appraisal of the literature, identifying knowledge gaps, and use of a particular theory to tie the work into what has already been published will continue to need the author's critical thinking skills. The essential social, emotional, and behavioral habits that support academic writing will remain at the core of being a successful author.

Our hope is that you find the resources in this book useful in moving your DNP project report forward to a publishable manuscript. We look forward to reading your publication!

# References

Castner, J., Amberson, T., Gillespie, G. L., & Douma, M. J. (2020). Deciding to post a manuscript preprint. *Nurse Author & Editor, 30*(4), 41–44. https://doi.org/10.1111/nae2.12

Fallon, L., Grapin, S., Newman, D. S., & Noltemeyer, A. (2022). Promoting equity and social justice in the peer review process: Tips for reviewers. *School Psychology International, 43*(1), 12–17. https://doi.org/10.1177/01430343211070165

Flanagin, A., Fontanarosa, P. B., & Bauchner, H. (2020). Preprints involving medical research—do the benefits outweigh the challenges? *JAMA, 324*(18), 1840–1843. https://doi.org/10.1001/jama.2020.20674

Hermanns, M., & Parker, C. (2020). Collaboration tools to enhance faculty productivity: Which one is right for your team? *Research and Theory for Nursing Practice, 34*(4), 289–292. https://doi.org/10.1891/RTNP-D-20-00110

International Committee of Medical Journal Editors. (2022). *Recommendations for conducting, reporting, editing, and publishing scholarly work in medical journals. Defining the role of authors and contributors.* https://www.icmje.org/recommendations/browse/roles-and-responsibilities/defining-the-role-of-authors-and-contributors.html

Johns Hopkins Medicine (2024). Johns Hopkins School of Medicine. Office of faculty development. Writing accountability groups (WAGS). https://www.hopkinsmedicine.org/faculty-development/career-path/wags

Merriam-Webster. (n.d.). *Curated.* https://www.merriam-webster.com/dictionary/curated

Millar, B. C., & Lim, M. (2022). The role of visual abstracts in the dissemination of medical research. *The Ulster Medical Journal, 91*(2), 67–78.

Mullins D. W. (2023). Instruction of content curation through learner-created infographics. *Medical Education, 57*(11), 1126. https://doi.org/10.1111/medu.15224

Oermann, M. H., & Nicoll, L. H. (2020). A primer on preprints. *Nurse Author & Editor, 30*(2), 1–10. https://doi.org/10.1111/j.1750-4910.2020.tb00564.x

Reed, J. M. (2023). Using generative AI to produce images for nursing education. *Nurse Educator, 48*(5), 246. https://doi.org/10.1097/NNE.0000000000001453

Rivkin, A. (2020). Manuscript referencing errors and their impact on shaping current evidence. *American Journal of Pharmaceutical Education, 84*(7). https://doi.org/10.5688/ajpe7846

Sallam, M. (2023). ChatGPT utility in healthcare education, research, and practice: Systematic review on the promising perspectives and valid concerns. *Healthcare, 11*(6), 887. https://doi.org/10.3390/healthcare11060887

Spicer, J. O., & Coleman, C. G. (2022). Creating effective infographics and visual abstracts to disseminate research and facilitate medical education on social media. *Clinical Infectious Diseases: An Official Publication of the Infectious Diseases Society of America, 74*(3), e14–e22. https://doi.org/10.1093/cid/ciac058

Springer. (2023, July). *Self archiving and sharing policies.* https://connect.springerpub.com/journal-article-sharing-policies

Sword, H. (2017). *Air & light & time & space: How successful academics write.* Harvard University Press.

Traboco, L., Pandian, H., Nikiphorou, E., & Gupta, L. (2022). Designing infographics: Visual representations for enhancing education, communication, and scientific research. *Journal of Korean Medical Science, 37*(27), e214. https://doi.org/10.3346/jkms.2022.37.e214

Watson, R. (2020). How to publish a preprint. A how-to on how to publish a preprint. *Nurse Author and Editor, 30*(2), 1–6.

Yarris, L. M., Artino Jr., A. R., Deiorio, N. M., Ten Cate, O., Sullivan, G. M., & Simpson, D. (2020). Envisioning the future of academic writing. *Journal of Graduate Medical Education, 12*(1), 1–6.

# INDEX